Gene Therapy

Other books in the Great Medical Discoveries series:

Cloning
Vaccines
Tuberculosis

Great Medical Discoveries

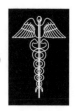

Gene Therapy

by Lisa Yount

On cover: Physician Robert Butz
conducts an experiment in gene therapy.

To Charlie:
Hope there'll soon be some good genes for you.

Library of Congress Cataloging-in-Publication Data

Yount, Lisa.
  Gene therapy /by Lisa Yount.
      p. cm. — (Great medical discoveries)
Includes bibliographical references and index.
Summary: Discusses the history of genetics, how knowledge of
genes has been developed to treat illnesses, and ethical issues
related to gene therapy.
  ISBN 1-56006-928-7
  1. Gene therapy—Juvenile literature. [1.Gene therapy. 2.
Genetics.] I. Title. II. Series.
  RB155 .8 .Y68 2002
  616'.042—dc21

2001003773

Copyright © 2002 by Lucent Books
an imprint of The Gale Group
10911 Technology Place, San Diego, CA 92127
Printed in the U.S.A.

CONTENTS

FOREWORD

Throughout history, people have struggled to understand and conquer the diseases and physical ailments that plague us. Once in a while, a discovery has changed the course of medicine and sometimes, the course of history itself. The stories of these discoveries have many elements in common—accidental findings, sudden insights, human dedication, and most of all, powerful results. Many illnesses that in the past were essentially a death warrant for their sufferers are today curable or even virtually extinct. And exciting new directions in medicine promise a future in which the building blocks of human life itself—the genes—may be manipulated and altered to restore health or to prevent disease from occurring in the first place.

It has been said that an insight is simply a rearrangement of already-known facts, and as often as not, these great medical discoveries have resulted partly from a reexamination of earlier efforts in light of new knowledge. Nineteenth-century monk Gregor Mendel experimented with pea plants for years, quietly unlocking the mysteries of genetics. However, the importance of his findings went unnoticed until three separate scientists, studying cell division with a newly improved invention called a microscope, rediscovered his work decades after his death. French doctor Jean-Antoine Villemin's experiments with rabbits proved that tuberculosis was contagious, but his conclusions were politely ignored by the medical community until another doctor, Robert Koch of Germany, discovered the exact culprit—the tubercle bacillus germ—years later.

Accident, too, has played a part in some medical discoveries. Because the tuberculosis germ does not stain with dye as easily as other bacteria, Koch was able to see it only after he had let a treated slide sit far longer than he intended. An unwanted speck of mold led Englishman Alexander Fleming to recognize the bacteria-killing qualities of the penicillium fungi, ushering in the era of antibiotic "miracle drugs."

That researchers sometimes benefited from fortuitous accidents does not mean that they were bumbling amateurs who relied solely on luck. They were dedicated scientists whose work created the conditions under which such lucky events could occur; many sacrificed years of their lives to observation and experimentation. Sometimes the price they paid was higher. Rene Launnec, who invented the stethoscope to help him study the effects of tuberculosis, himself succumbed to the disease.

And humanity has benefited from these scientists' efforts. The formerly terrifying disease of smallpox has been eliminated from the face of the earth—the only case of the complete conquest of a once deadly disease. Tuberculosis, perhaps the oldest disease known to humans and certainly one of its most prolific killers, has been essentially wiped out in some parts of the world. Genetically engineered insulin is a godsend to countless diabetics who are allergic to the animal insulin that has traditionally been used to help them.

Despite such triumphs there are few unequivocal success stories in the history of great medical discoveries. New strains of tuberculosis are proving to be resistant to the antibiotics originally developed to treat them, raising the specter of a resurgence of the disease that has killed 2 billion people over the course of human history. But medical research continues on numerous fronts and will no doubt lead to still undreamed-of advancements in the future.

Each volume in the Great Medical Discoveries series tells the story of one great medical breakthrough—the first gropings for understanding, the pieces that came together and how, and the immediate and longer-term results. Part science and part social history, the series explains some of the key findings that have shaped modern medicine and relieved untold human suffering. Numerous primary and secondary source quotations enhance the text and bring to life all the drama of scientific discovery. Sidebars highlight personalities and convey personal stories. The series also discusses the future of each medical discovery—a future in which vaccines may guard against AIDS, gene therapy may eliminate cancer, and other as-yet unimagined treatments may become commonplace.

INTRODUCTION

Gene Therapy: A New Medical Frontier

Alexandra Fyodorovna was czarina, or empress, of Russia, and the wealth and power of a huge country was hers to command. All she wanted, however, was to make her child well. Every time he had the slightest scratch or bruise, her only son, Czarevitch (Crown Prince) Alexis, bled and bled. (A bruise is actually bleeding under the skin, caused by bumping or hitting something.) Several times he almost died from such injuries. No doctor could help him.

In 1905, two years after the frail prince's birth, a wild-looking man who called himself Rasputin appeared at the Russian court. He claimed that he was a holy man and could save the crown prince. Because of that claim, the desperate Alexandra and her husband, Czar Nicholas, gave Rasputin valuable gifts. As the years went on, he gained increasing power at court. Rasputin's claim was false and he abused his privilege, but the royal couple would never admit that he did anything wrong. Their dependence on him and willingness to take his advice about running the country contributed to the Russian people's growing anger with the czar's government. It was one cause of the revolution that

Crown Prince Alexis
inherited hemophilia,
the "royal disease,"
from his mother,
Czarina Alexandra.

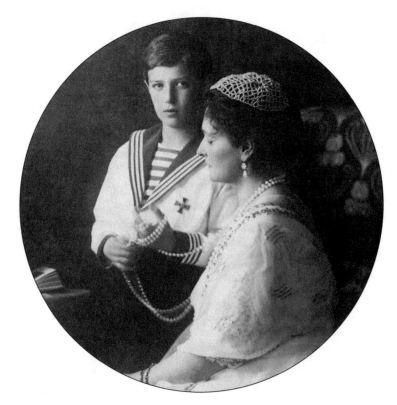

swept the country in 1917 and cost the royal family
their lives.

Crown Prince Alexis had a disease called hemophilia. People with this illness are born without a
substance that normally makes blood clot, or form a
sticky mass, soon after being released from a wound.
Without this substance, the blood keeps flowing, so a
hemophiliac can bleed to death from even a small
injury.

The prince's illness was a deadly, if unintended,
legacy from the very mother who wanted so badly to
cure it. Alexandra, although healthy herself, carried
its seeds within her body and passed them on to her
son. So many other boys in her large family, descendants of Britain's Queen Victoria, had the same sickness that it came to be known as the "royal disease."
Observant physicians had known for at least seven-
teen hundred years that hemophilia was inherited.

Gene Defects

Few cases of inherited illness have had as much effect on history as Crown Prince Alexis's did, but such sicknesses have caused untold heartbreak for individual families. Some four thousand inherited diseases are known today. Twentieth-century scientists have learned that these sicknesses are caused by defects in genes, chemical units carrying coded information that acts like a blueprint or computer program to shape an individual's life. Most living things receive half their genes from their mother and half from their father. Every microscopic cell in their bodies carries a copy of these genes. A human being's genome, or complete genetic collection, contains 30,000 to 100,000 genes.

Genes' contribution to disease does not end with obviously inherited diseases like hemophilia. Scientists have discovered that subtle defects in genes make certain people more likely than average to develop much more common diseases, such as cancer and heart disease. "Researchers have concluded that virtually all human illness . . . has some relationship to genetic endowment,"[1] Pulitzer prize–winning *Chicago Tribune* reporters Jeff Lyon and Peter Gorner write.

Even today, when medicine can cure many illnesses that once were fatal, there is little treatment for most inherited diseases and no cure for any of them. For example, a woman who has inherited a high likelihood of developing breast cancer, a non-inherited disease influenced by genes, can do little about it except have frequent tests to spot the disease in its early stages, when chances of successful treatment are greatest.

This is starting to change, however. Researchers have learned a great deal about what genes are and how they affect health. They have identified the genetic defects that lead to hemophilia and many other inherited diseases or that make some people likely to develop other illnesses such as cancer. Even more important, they are beginning to be able to change genes in ways that restore health. In some cases, they try to replace genes that are missing or damaged. In others, they add genes to make the body produce substances that fight disease.

Gene therapy—altering genes to treat or prevent disease—is one of the most exciting frontiers of medicine today. Its supporters believe that in the twenty-first century it will revolutionize the treatment of illness as completely as antibiotics did in the twentieth century. Leroy Hood, a scientist who developed new ways to identify genes, predicted in 1995 that "over the next twenty to forty years, we will have the potential for eradicating [wiping out] the major diseases that plague the American population"[2] by means of gene therapy.

Critics, however, say that claims for gene therapy's power have been exaggerated. They point out that it has yet to cure a single person. They say that some tests of gene therapy have been carried out in a way that needlessly endangered patients' lives. Their complaints show how much scientists still need to learn before gene therapy can fulfill its promise. Furthermore, both supporters and opponents agree that even if gene therapy becomes as widely used as its advocates expect, it will raise troubling ethical questions for scientists and ordinary citizens alike.

CHAPTER 1

Deadly Legacies

People have been choosing and changing genes since the beginning of human history. Farmers did it when they saved seeds from the best plants in one year's crop to plant in the following year. Ranchers did it when they let only their strongest and most productive animals mate and bear offspring. Men and women did it when they chose mates who looked energetic and healthy. To be sure, none of these people had ever heard of a gene. All they knew was that offspring tended to be like their parents. By selecting parents, people could eventually, over many generations, produce offspring with features they wanted.

Natural Selection

In the mid–nineteenth century, British naturalist Charles Darwin revolutionized biology by saying that nature did the same thing plant and animal breeders did. Living things of the same type, or species, were similar to each other, Darwin said, but individuals within a species still varied in small ways. For example, a deer might happen to be born with slightly more powerful leg muscles than others of its kind, allowing it to run faster. The extra speed might increase this particular deer's chance of escaping predators and, therefore, living long enough to have offspring. Chances are good that at least some of the

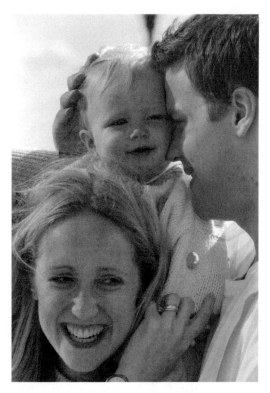

Genes pass traits and characteristics from parent to child.

deer's offspring would inherit its unusual leg muscles and, in turn, have a better chance to reproduce.

In this way, Darwin maintained, nature "bred" living things to develop and preserve characteristics that helped them survive in the environments where they lived. He called his theory "evolution by natural selection." Evolution is the slow change in types of living things over time, and natural selection is the mechanism that Darwin proposed as the cause of this change. Other thinkers had suggested that life might evolve, but Darwin was the first to suggest a believable process through which these changes could come about.

Darwin knew his theory depended on the fact that parents somehow passed characteristics, or traits, on to their offspring, yet he had no idea how this was done. He also knew that heredity was unpredictable, but neither he nor most other biologists of his time understood why. In his groundbreaking book *On the Origin of Species by Means of Natural Selection*, published in 1859, Darwin admitted:

> No one can say why the same peculiarity [trait] in different individuals . . . is sometimes inherited and sometimes not so; why the child often reverts in certain characters to [has certain characteristics resembling] its grandfather, or other more remote ancestor; why a peculiarity is often transmitted from one sex to both sexes, or to one sex alone.[3]

Mathematics in a Garden

Darwin never learned that, perhaps while he was writing those very words, a quiet man in a monastery garden in what is now the Czech Republic was working out the solution to the puzzle Darwin described. Over a period of eight years this man, a monk named Gregor Mendel, grew thousands of pea plants with eight well-defined characteristics, such as height and seed color. By counting the number of offspring with different forms of these traits in each generation, Mendel learned that the traits were passed on in patterns that could be described by simple mathematical rules.

One trait that Mendel studied was the shape that pea seeds took after they had dried out. The seeds of

Shocking Ideas

Charles Darwin's On the Origin of Species *deeply distressed many people of his time. In his book on the history of genetics,* The Engineer in the Garden, *British science writer Colin Tudge explains one reason for this shock:*

To them, each "species" was an ideal, . . . God's fundamental vision of what their particular type should be like. . . . What really offended critics was Darwin's insistence that one species could change into another, or—even worse—that one species could

Evolutionist and naturalist Charles Darwin.

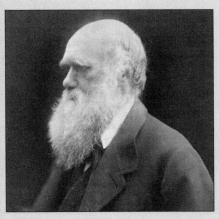

diverge [split off] to form several, or even thousands of new species.

Today most people accept the idea that species can change naturally. However, some object to humans' direct alteration of genes, often called genetic engineering, for much the same reason that their ancestors objected to Darwin's ideas—except that, ironically, evolution has replaced God as the power that should not be defied. For example, in the September 2000 Hastings Center Report, *British philosopher Mary Midgley writes in an essay titled "Biotechnology and Monstrosity: Why We Should Pay Attention to the 'Yuk Factor'":*

Our [mythological and scientific] tradition has so far held that . . . the boundaries of a species should be respected. . . . Any change [in a species] that is not directly demanded by altered outside circumstances is likely to be lethal [deadly]. Evolution . . . knows what it is about [what it is doing] when it puts together the repertoire [collection] of characteristics that marks a species.

Some people fear that changing human genes, as gene therapy proposes to do, eventually will alter the nature of the human species.

some plants remained smooth and round, while the seeds of others shriveled and became wrinkled. Mendel knew that these characteristics could be dependably inherited. Smooth-seeded plants mated with other smooth-seeded plants always produced offspring with smooth seeds, and the same was true of wrinkled-seeded plants.

When Mendel bred a smooth-seeded plant with a wrinkled-seeded one, however, something strange happened: All the offspring had smooth seeds. Where had the wrinkled type of seed gone? The answer showed itself when he mated these first-generation hybrids (offspring of parents that differ from each other in some characteristic) with one another. Carefully counting the results of many such experiments, Mendel found that he had obtained 5,474 round-seeded plants and 1,850 wrinkled-seeded ones. In other words, an average of three out of every four of these second-generation plants produced smooth seeds, while the fourth had wrinkled seeds.

By studying pea plants and their offspring, Gregor Mendel discovered how traits are inherited.

Mendel concluded that inherited traits were controlled by something he called factors, which were passed from parents to offspring. A living thing inherited one factor determining each trait from its male parent and one from its female parent. Factors for some forms of a trait, such as smooth seeds in peas, seemed to be more powerful than others. Mendel termed these forms dominant. Forms of a trait that were weaker, such as wrinkled seeds, he called recessive—likely to recede, or pull back. If a living thing inherited a factor for the dominant form of a trait from one parent and a factor for the recessive form of the trait from the other parent, the monk decided, the dominant form would always show itself.

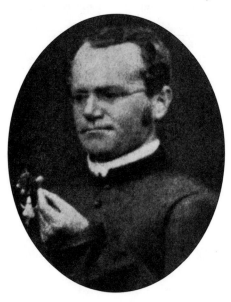

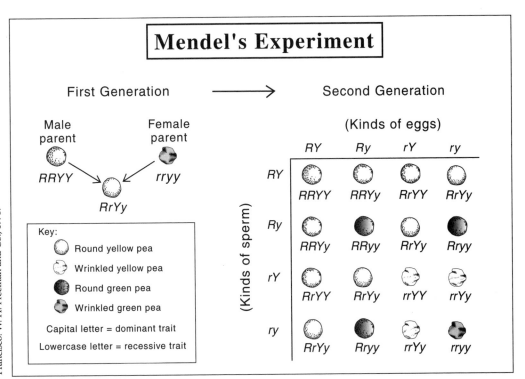

Source: Sam Singer and Henry R. Hilgard, *The Biology of People*. San Francisco: W. H. Freeman and Co., 1978.

The factor carrying the recessive form, however, still existed and could be passed on to that living thing's offspring. The recessive form would appear only in living things that had inherited the recessive factor from both parents.

Mendel published the results of his experiments in the journal of the Natural History Society of Brünn (now Brno), the city where his monastery was located, in 1866. Although copies went to many university libraries in Europe, few scientists apparently read Mendel's paper. Fewer still realized that the monk's tedious-looking mathematics had an importance that reached far beyond the breeding of garden plants. Mendel died, still unappreciated by science, in 1884.

The Birth of Genetics

Only in 1900, when three different scientists independently rediscovered Mendel's work, did researchers begin to understand that he had laid out the basic rules of inheritance for nearly all living things. Furthermore, he had supplied the missing piece in Darwin's theory of evolution by showing how traits favored by natural selection could be passed on. In 1909 Wilhelm Johannsen, one of the scientists who studied Mendel's paper, changed the monk's term *factors* to *genes*, from a Latin root meaning "race" or "type." Thus the science of genetics—the study of the mechanisms by which traits are passed on from parents to offspring—was born.

Once the idea of genes had been proposed, it did not take scientists long to suggest that genes might lie at the root of some diseases. Most people knew of some family in which a certain kind of illness cropped up much more often, and perhaps earlier in life, than it did in the general population. Farmers had noticed that plants or animals in certain lines of descent did not thrive as well as others or tended to develop certain kinds of problems.

The first person to show that a particular disease was inherited was an English physician named Archibald Garrod. Garrod, working with William Bateson, a pioneer of genetics, studied a rare condition called alkaptonuria. The bodies of people with this disease cannot break down a chemical called homogentisic acid. The chemical passes out in their urine and makes the urine turn black when it is exposed to air. The black urine does them no harm, but the same defect makes them likely to suffer from the painful joint disease called arthritis.

In 1902, Garrod and Bateson showed that alkaptonuria ran in families. In other words, people with the disease always had close relatives who also had it. Furthermore, both parents of a child with alkaptonuria always came from families in which the disease occurred.

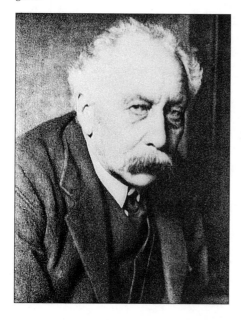

Genetics pioneer William Bateson concluded that the disease alkaptonuria was probably inherited through a recessive gene.

(In fact they often came from the same family. Parents of children with the disease were frequently first cousins, which meant that they carried many of the same genes.) On average, too, one out of four of the children of two such people had the disease. This was the same pattern that Mendel had shown for inheritance of recessive traits in his garden peas. Garrod and Bateson concluded, therefore, that alkaptonuria was probably caused by a recessive gene.

Inside the Cell

At first, the pioneers of genetics had little more idea than Mendel about what, physically, factors—or genes—are. They gained some clues, however, from discoveries that the improved microscopes invented in the mid–nineteenth century had allowed scientists to make about cells, the microscopic building blocks of which all living things are made. Most cells, these researchers had found, contain a smaller body called the nucleus. Inside the nucleus the scientists saw material that became colored when the cell was treated with a certain type of dye. Walther Flemming, the German scientist who discovered this substance in 1875, called it chromatin, from a Greek word meaning "color." Just before a cell divided, the chromatin formed itself into pairs of threadlike bodies that another scientist named chromosomes. Cells of different species proved to have different numbers of chromosomes. Humans, for instance, have forty-six, arranged in twenty-three pairs.

By the time Mendel's work was rediscovered, much evidence suggested that chromosomes behaved exactly as would be predicted if they were (or carried) Mendel's factors. For instance, the sex cells (sperm in males and eggs in females), which combined to make a new living thing, proved to contain half as many chromosomes as other body cells. This would be expected; otherwise, the number of chromosomes (factors, or genes) an offspring inherits would double in each generation.

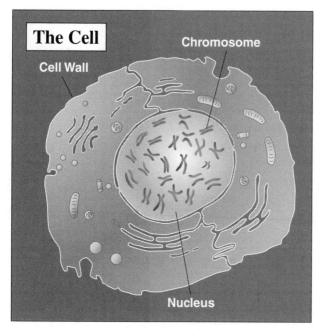

The Cell

Cell Wall

Chromosome

Nucleus

In 1903 a young American scientist, Walter Sutton, became the first to clearly propose that factors were a physical part of chromosomes. Because living things had far fewer chromosomes than they had characteristics, it seemed clear that each chromosome must contain a number of factors, or genes. The evidence supporting the chromosome theory was all indirect, however. A number of geneticists therefore doubted the idea at first.

Fruit Flies and Chromosomes

Proof of the chromosome theory—and much more information about genes—came from the study of fruit flies, creatures much less pleasant than Mendel's peas. Thomas Hunt Morgan's laboratory at Columbia University in New York City was packed with bottles full of the tiny, buzzing insects. Morgan and his coworkers and students found the flies to be ideal genetic test subjects because they were smallz and easy to raise, reproduced in great numbers, and took only about ten days to grow up. The insects also had many traits, such as different colors of eyes and shapes of wings, that were easy to identify under a magnifying glass and were inherited according to Mendel's rules.

In 1910 one of Morgan's students spotted a fly with a white eye. This was unusual, because most fruit flies' eyes are red. Morgan knew that the white eye had to be caused by a mutation, or change, in a gene that controlled eye color. (Mutations, which usually occur by chance, are one of the main sources of the variations within species that are so important in Darwin's theory.) Morgan mated the white-eyed fly, a male, with a normal, red-eyed female. All their offspring had red eyes, which showed that the white-eye gene was recessive. The next generation bred from these flies showed Mendel's classic three-to-one inheritance ratio, with one exception: All the white-eyed flies were male. This fact provided a vital clue about the eye-color gene's location.

Source: Colin Tudge, The Engineer in the Garden: Genes ansd Genetics: From the Idea of Heredity to the Creation of Life. London: Jonathan Cape, 1993.

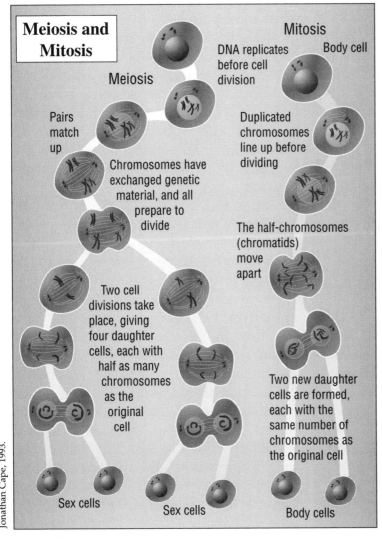

Meiosis and Mitosis

Mitosis

Meiosis

DNA replicates before cell division

Body cell

Pairs match up

Duplicated chromosomes line up before dividing

Chromosomes have exchanged genetic material, and all prepare to divide

The half-chromosomes (chromatids) move apart

Two cell divisions take place, giving four daughter cells, each with half as many chromosomes as the original cell

Two new daughter cells are formed, each with the same number of chromosomes as the original cell

Sex cells

Sex cells

Body cells

In 1905 geneticists Nettie Stevens and Edmund Wilson had noticed that in males of most animal species (including fruit flies and humans), one pair of chromosomes—unlike all the others—consists of two chromosomes that look quite different. The larger of these is called the X chromosome, and the smaller is the Y. Females have two X chromosomes, but males have an X and a Y. This pair of chromosomes thus determines an offspring's sex. Every child inherits an X chromosome from its mother, so living things are male only if they inherit a Y chromosome, rather than an X, from their male parent.

Because females have two X chromosomes, their cells have two copies of all genes carried on the X chromosome. Males, however, have only one X chromosome and, therefore, one copy of these genes. If a female inherits one dominant gene and one recessive gene for a trait such as eye color, Mendel's rules say that she will show the dominant form of the trait. She may, however, pass either the dominant or the recessive gene on to her offspring. If a recessive gene is on the X chromosome and a male inherits it from his mother, he will show the recessive form of the trait because he will receive no other gene from his father to cancel it out. This seemed to be what was happening with the white-eyed fruit flies. Morgan concluded in 1911, therefore, that the gene that determined the flies' eye color must be on the X chromosome.

The fruit-fly eye-color gene was the first gene, other than the one that determines sex, that was shown to be carried on a particular chromosome. Morgan's discovery helped to convince him and others that the chromosome theory was correct. Certain other recessive genes, including the one that causes hemophilia (the disease that made Crown Prince Alexis so

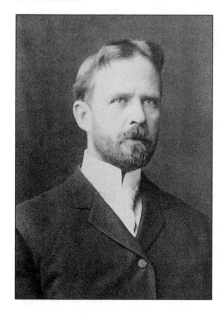

Thomas Hunt Morgan determined that the gene determining the eye color of a fruit fly is based on the X chromosome.

sick), were later found to show themselves almost entirely in males. They, too, were likely to be carried on the X chromosome.

Nucleic Acid or Protein?

Proving that genes were carried on chromosomes did not settle the question of what genes actually were. Scientists knew that genes had to be some form of chemical, because cells are made up of chemicals. They also realized that the structure of this chemical had to convey inherited information in a coded form, just as the letters of an alphabet, arranged in different ways, provide a code for the words and ideas of a language. They assumed that a chemical could carry complicated information only if the chemical itself was complex, made up of many simpler substances. They could not believe that a genetic "alphabet" with only a handful of letters could spell out enough different pieces of information to specify all the traits that a plant or animal possesses.

Biochemists in the late nineteenth century had found out that chromosomes contain two kinds of chemicals: proteins and nucleic acids. Proteins are a large family of substances, and scientists knew that the structure and chemistry of cells depend on them. The membranes that surround cells contain proteins, for instance. Other proteins, called enzymes, control the speed of chemical reactions in the cell. Many of the substances taking part in those reactions are also proteins. Much less had been discovered about nucleic acids. Researchers knew that there were two types: deoxyribonucleic acid, or DNA, and ribonucleic acid, or RNA. However, they had not found out what work nucleic acids did in cells.

In 1941 two scientists at California's Stanford University showed that genes produce traits by somehow directing the making of proteins. After that, researchers redefined a gene as a piece of inherited information that controls the making of one protein.

Furthermore, many geneticists thought that genes themselves would turn out to be proteins. The chief reason for this belief was that proteins are complex molecules made up of twenty types of molecules called amino acids. That seemed to be more than enough "letters" for a genetic alphabet, even though an individual protein normally does not contain all twenty kinds of amino acids. Nucleic acids, by contrast, contain only four kinds of smaller molecules that seemed likely to act as parts of a hereditary code. These molecules are called bases. (Nucleic acids also contain molecules of phosphate and sugar, but the amounts of these substances do not vary in different molecules of nucleic acid, so scientists concluded that they probably were not part of the genetic code.)

A New York scientist named Oswald Avery gave believers in the protein theory a major surprise in 1944. Avery worked with two types, or strains, of bacteria called pneumococcus. One form of pneumococcus could cause lung disease in mice, whereas another was unable to produce illness. Bacteria with the power to cause sickness could pass this ability on to their descendants, so it had to be carried in their genes.

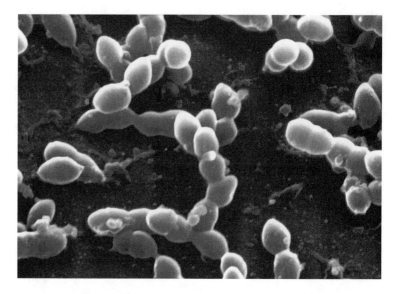

Scientist Oswald Avery proved that DNA carries inherited information through his studies of bacteria called pneumococcus (pictured).

When Avery mixed pneumococcus bacteria that could not cause sickness with dead bacteria of the disease-causing kind, the living bacteria suddenly became able to make mice sick. Their offspring also showed this power. It was clear, therefore, that the living bacteria had taken up or absorbed something from the dead ones that had changed their genes. Avery showed that this could happen when the dead bacteria had been treated with a substance that dissolved protein but not when they were treated with a chemical that destroyed DNA. This meant that DNA had to be the material that contained the inherited information.

The Double Helix

Scientists who studied genes now realized that they needed to learn more about the structure of DNA. Finding out how the small molecules that make up DNA are arranged inside the large DNA molecule would give the researchers valuable clues about the way DNA reproduces itself, as genetic material has to do in order to be able to be passed on to descendants, and the way it encodes inherited information. Three groups of scientists began racing to make this important discovery.

The winners of the race were two researchers working at Britain's prestigious Cambridge University. One was a young American named James Watson, the other the somewhat older Englishman Francis Crick. Watson and Crick worked with models of molecules, which they assembled like a scientist's version of Tinkertoys. They also studied X-ray photographs of nucleic acid molecules made by another British scientist, Rosalind Franklin. From evidence in these two sources, they concluded that the DNA molecule had to have a shape that they called a double helix.

DNA's double helix is like a spiral staircase or a twisted ladder. Its sides are made up of phosphate and sugar molecules. Its steps, or rungs, consist of

Using a model, James Watson (left) and Francis Crick demonstrate how a DNA double helix, which looks like a twisted ladder, reproduces itself.

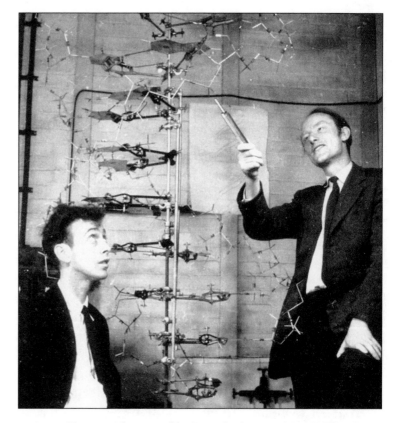

pairs of bases chemically bonded together. DNA contains four types of bases: adenine (abbreviated A), cytosine (C), guanine (G), and thymine (T). Watson and Crick worked out that adenine always pairs with thymine, and cytosine always pairs with guanine

Watson and Crick published a short paper describing their picture of the DNA molecule in the British science magazine *Nature* on April 25, 1953. It concluded with the understated sentence, "It has not escaped our notice that the specific pairing we have postulated [proposed] immediately suggests a possible copying mechanism for the genetic material."[4] Crick was less understated when he wrote to his son, "We think we have found the basic mechanism by which life comes from life."[5]

Five weeks later the two scientists published a second paper that explained the statement with which they ended their first one. When a cell is preparing to divide, they said, the chemical bonds holding the pairs of bases together break down. The DNA double helix then splits apart lengthwise like a zipper unzipping. Free-floating units, each consisting of a base and an attached piece of phosphate-sugar "backbone," attach themselves to each half to create the same pattern as had existed before. The result is two DNA molecules just like the original one. When a cell divides, creating two "daughter" cells, one copy of each DNA molecule goes to one daughter cell and the other copy goes to the other cell. Experiments proved this theory correct in 1958.

The Genetic Code

During the late 1950s and early 1960s, Crick and others went on to figure out how DNA carries the information that does the genes' main job: telling a cell how to make proteins. Crick, among others, guessed from the beginning that the information must somehow be encoded in the order, or sequence, of the bases inside the long DNA molecule, because this is the only feature that varies from one DNA molecule to another. At first, however, no one could see how just four bases could represent twenty amino acids. This was the same puzzle that had kept many earlier scientists from believing that nucleic acids could contain inherited information. Units of two bases would not work, because they allow only 16 (4 x 4) combinations, not enough to stand for all the amino acids. Crick pointed out in 1957, though, that units made up of three bases would provide 64 (4 x 4 x 4) combinations, more than enough to do the job. With that many choices, several different three-based combinations probably stood for each amino acid.

Crick and another Cambridge scientist, Sydney Brenner, proved this triplet theory in 1961. A number of laboratories then began racing to decipher what came to be called the genetic code, determining which of the sixty-four possible combinations of three bases

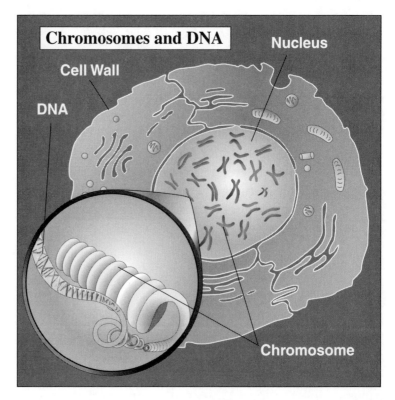

Chromosomes and DNA · Nucleus · Cell Wall · DNA · Chromosome

stood for which amino acids. This work was completed by 1966. Scientists also worked out the details of the complex process by which a stretch of DNA with a certain sequence of bases—a gene—produces a protein containing a certain sequence of amino acids.

By about 1970 geneticists and molecular biologists had learned a great deal about genes. They had a good idea of what genes were, what they did, and how they did it. They also knew that certain diseases occurred in families and were passed on in the patterns Mendel had described, which meant that these illnesses were almost surely caused by defects in genes. A few farsighted scientists had even begun to predict that someday it might be possible to treat these diseases by repairing or replacing the damaged genes. No one had any idea, however, how this might be done.

CHAPTER 2

The Birth of Gene Therapy

Greek legend tells of a fire-breathing monster called a chimera. This fearsome patchwork beast—part dragon, part goat, and part lion—terrorized the countryside until a hero destroyed it.

In the mid-1970s many people were equally terrified to find out that scientists had begun making chimeras of their own. These new creatures, containing genes from different kinds of living things, were so small that they could be seen only with a microscope. Still, popular thinking—and the thinking of some scientists as well—held that they might turn out to be monsters all the same. A few people, however, hoped they would prove to be angels in disguise.

Gene Splicers

California scientists led the way in developing what came to be called gene-splicing, recombinant DNA technology, or genetic engineering: artificially combining genes from different species of living things. Paul Berg of Stanford University, near San Francisco, was probably the first gene splicer. He prepared genes for combining by treating DNA from different living things with chemicals called restriction enzymes, which come

29

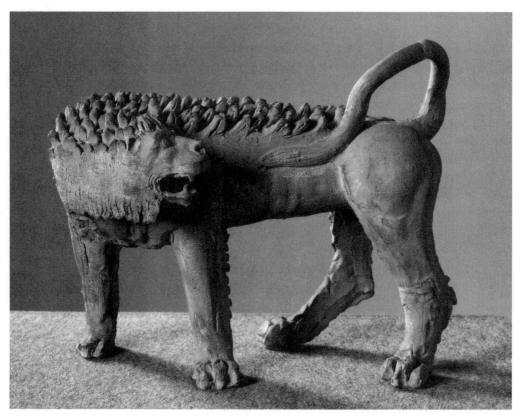

In the mid-1970s, scientists learned how to splice genes together to create living things with characteristics of more than one species, like the mythical Greek monster called the chimera.

from bacteria. These substances act like molecular scissors, cutting DNA apart at any spot where they find a certain sequence of bases. Different bacteria have different restriction enzymes, and each kind snips DNA at a different sequence. The enzymes can cut any DNA, no matter what kind of living thing it comes from.

Berg took advantage of the fact that restriction enzymes break the two strands of a DNA molecule unevenly, leaving "sticky ends"—pieces of single-stranded DNA a few bases long. The short, single-stranded piece at one end of each long, double-stranded DNA stretch has a base sequence exactly opposite to that at the other end. If, for instance, one end has the sequence T-A-C-G, the other end will have the sequence G-C-A-T. Each of these pieces of single-stranded DNA chemically attracts bases in the reverse sequence, just as they would if the DNA was reproducing. Any piece of

DNA ending in that sequence, therefore, will join with the sticky end.

All pieces of DNA treated with the same restriction enzyme will have the same pairs of mirror-image sticky ends. This means that, for example, a DNA fragment from a bacterium and one from a mouse that have been treated with the same enzyme will both end in T-A-C-G on one side and G-C-A-T on the other. This allows the two pieces of DNA to be joined or spliced together because the G-C-A-T end of the mouse DNA will stick to the T-A-C-G end of the bacteria DNA, and vice versa. In 1972 Berg treated DNA from two kinds of viruses with the same restriction enzyme and then joined the resulting fragments together. He thus made the first pieces of DNA that contained genetic material from two different types of living things.

Hints of Danger

Berg next intended to put DNA from a virus called SV40, which causes cancer in monkeys, into a living bacterium. He planned to use a common type of bacterium called *Escherichia coli* (*E. coli* for short) in this experiment. *E. coli* lives in the human intestine and is usually harmless. When another scientist, Robert Pollack, heard about Berg's plan, however, he persuaded Berg not to carry it out. Putting genes from a cancer-causing virus into a bacterium that normally infects humans could be dangerous, Pollack said. What if some of the altered bacteria escaped from the laboratory and proved able to cause cancers in people?

After thinking about it, Berg decided that Pollack was right. He not only stopped his own SV40 experiments but called on other scientists to stop recombinant DNA research involving bacteria or viruses that might prove dangerous

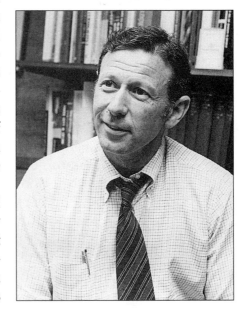

Paul Berg produced the first pieces of DNA containing genetic material from two different types of living things.

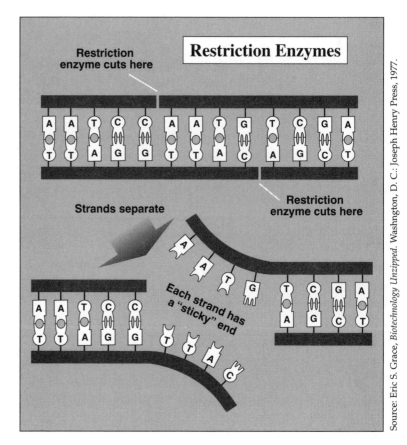

Source: Eric S. Grace, *Biotechnology Unzipped*. Washington, D. C.: Joseph Henry Press, 1977.

until steps to increase safety could be taken. When word of the scientists' concerns reached the media, many nonscientists also demanded a halt to possibly dangerous gene-splicing experiments. Some wanted genetic engineering banned altogether.

On October 17, 1974, in response to this concern, the National Institutes of Health (NIH) established a group called the Recombinant DNA Advisory Committee, or RAC. The RAC, composed of both scientists and nonscientists, was supposed to review and approve plans for all genetic engineering experiments before the experiments took place. In 1976 the NIH also published safety guidelines for laboratories doing gene-splicing research. These guidelines were intended to make sure no altered microbes that might be dangerous could escape.

Microscopic Workhorses

Despite public fears, genetic engineering moved ahead rapidly. In 1973, while Berg and Pollack were talking about halting Berg's experiments, another Stanford scientist took gene-splicing further, though in a less dangerous direction. This scientist, Stanley Cohen, worked with Herbert Boyer, a researcher at the University of California's San Francisco campus. Using the same restriction enzyme Berg had employed, Cohen and Boyer snipped a piece of DNA

Safety Conference by the Sea

In an article titled "Lessons from Asilomar," published in Science News *on February 23, 1985, Julie Ann Miller describes the conference at which scientists had hammered out safety rules for the then-new technique of gene-splicing ten years before.*

Among redwoods, Monterey pines and migrating monarch butterflies, 140 molecular biologists spent four long and intense days a decade ago. . . . The meeting in February 1975 at the Asilomar Conference Center in Pacific Grove, Calif., was unique in the history of biology. The scientists convened . . . to assess potential risks of the new technique and to suggest limitations of its use in research. The foremost risk then imagined was that a novel microorganism might be created experimentally—and released accidentally—to cause an epidemic of cancer or some new and incurable disease. The way the scientists dealt with such hypothetical [speculative] risks at that meeting continues to affect the conduct of biological research today. . . .

The meeting's organizers . . . recommended a scale of special safety procedures corresponding to a scale of conjectural [possible] hazards associated with different types of recombinant DNA experiments. . . . The majority at the meeting agreed, or at least did not vocally disagree, to the committee's recommendations. The [meeting's] report . . . became the basis of the National Institutes of Health (NIH) guidelines that have governed gene-splicing research throughout the United States since 1976. . . .

[Paul Berg says,] "At Asilomar we agreed that we didn't know enough to make a judgment [on the safety of gene-splicing], and 95 percent of us agreed that it would be better to go slow." [But] many scientists have objected . . . to the way the . . . meeting was run. . . . The important decisions . . . were made at the end of the meeting and the participants were allowed only to approve or reject, not to thoroughly discuss, the proposals. "All of us were tired," [Waclaw Szybalski of the University of Wisconsin] says. "It was the end, and we wanted to go home."

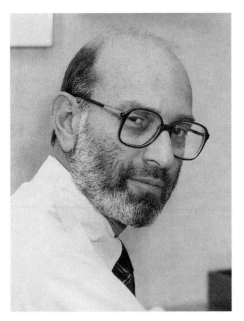

Stanley Cohen (pictured) and Herbert Boyer proved that a transferred gene could continue to make protein in its new location.

out of the genome of an African clawed toad and transferred it into *E. coli* bacteria. They went beyond Berg by showing that the transferred gene could make its protein in its new location. It could also be passed on to new generations of bacteria.

E. coli and other bacteria became genetic engineering's workhorses. Some scientists turned them into miniature factories to make proteins that were useful in medicine. In 1976, for instance, Herbert Boyer joined forces with venture capitalist Robert Swanson to form Genentech, probably the first company built around recombinant DNA technology. Their first product, sold beginning in 1982, was insulin, a protein that people with the common disease called diabetes must take throughout their lives to control their bodies' use of sugar. Insulin for diabetics had formerly come from the bodies of slaughtered cattle and pigs. Some diabetics, however, were allergic to animal insulin, which is slightly different from the human form. Genentech's insulin avoided this problem because it was essentially a human protein, churned out by bacteria containing the human insulin gene.

Other researchers used bacteria to help them identify particular genes. At first, gene identification was a complex and tedious process. Researchers used restriction enzymes to cut DNA into pieces and inserted the pieces into bacteria. Each gene-carrying bacterium was allowed to multiply into a colony, copying or cloning the foreign DNA every time it reproduced. The scientists then studied the colonies to see what proteins they made. Later decades brought great improvements in this technology, and today it can be carried out quickly and automatically by machines. The same is true of techniques for working out the order or sequence of bases within each gene, which reveals the sequence of amino acids in the protein the gene makes. Knowing the amino acid sequence helps scientists identify proteins and learn how they work.

Curing with Genes

By the late 1970s a few bold physician-researchers were beginning to think about using genetic engineering to treat disease. Scientists had learned how to transfer genes into the cells of complex living things as well as into bacteria. Many inherited diseases appeared to be caused by a mutation in a single gene, and family studies had shown that most of these damaged genes were recessive. If a normal copy of such a gene could be put into the cells that needed it, the researchers reasoned, the disease might be cured. This was the basic idea behind gene therapy.

The scientists' first choices for treatment were a group of diseases that cause problems in the blood. Each disease results from a single mistake in one of the several genes that carry the code for hemoglobin, the

Escherichia coli *became a workhorse for genetic engineering.*

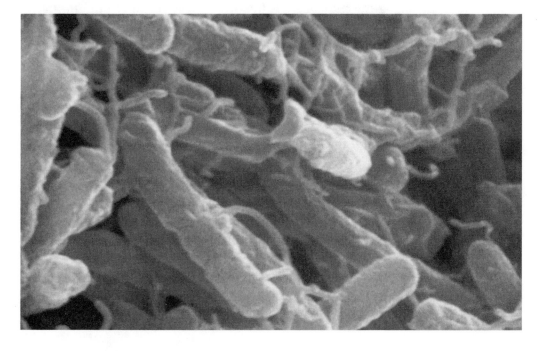

protein that gives blood its red color and transports life-giving oxygen throughout the body. (Geneticists had learned that several genes sometimes specify different parts of a single protein.) The hemoglobin genes were among the small number that had been identified, so the researchers knew which genes would have to be transferred. Furthermore, they knew that the genes would not have to be put into all the body's cells—an impossible task then and now. They needed only to get the genes into long-lived cells in the bone marrow (the soft, reddish substance inside certain bones) that make blood cells.

Most researchers hoped to use viruses as "delivery trucks" to carry healthy genes into cells. A virus is nothing more than a molecule of DNA or RNA, usually containing just a handful of genes, wrapped in a protein coat. It cannot reproduce on its own. Instead, it injects its genetic material into a cell. The material makes its way into the cell's nucleus and forces the cell to copy it, using the same procedure that the cell uses for copying its own DNA. If a healthy human gene had been spliced into a virus's genetic material, scientists expected that this gene would be inserted into the nucleus along with the virus's own genes when the virus invaded a cell. There, like other genes, it could function to make proteins.

Viruses can cause serious diseases such as rabies (the rabies virus is pictured), but scientists hoped to make certain viruses harmless and use them to inject healthy genes into cells.

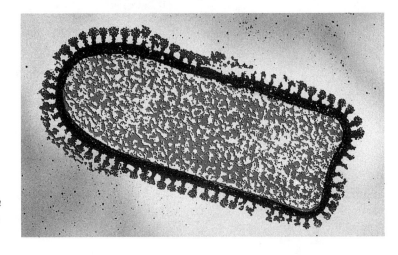

Normally, a virus forces a cell to make many copies of both its genetic material and its protein coat—in short, many new viruses. These viruses then burst out of the cell, killing it in the process, and go on to attack other cells. When many cells are destroyed, the result is disease. In order to use viruses in gene therapy, scientists needed to find a way to keep the viruses from reproducing and killing cells.

Richard Mulligan, then a graduate student in Paul Berg's laboratory, took the first step toward making viruses usable for gene therapy in 1979. He removed the genes from SV40 that made it able to reproduce and, in their place, inserted a hemoglobin gene from rabbits. He then mixed the altered virus with monkey cells in laboratory dishes. Mulligan showed that the engineered virus entered, or infected, some of the cells but did not harm them. Furthermore, the cells that had been infected became able to make the rabbit protein. This was the first time anyone had moved a gene from one kind of mammal into the cells of another and proved that the gene could function in its new home.

Only a small percentage of the cells in the dishes became infected, however. If this proved to be true of viruses carrying healthy genes into humans, the treatment might not affect enough bone marrow cells to cure or lessen the disease. No one knew whether such a treatment would be safe, either. It was possible that altered viruses might somehow regain their power to reproduce and kill cells after they had entered a human body or that they might damage cells in some way that the laboratory tests did not reveal.

A Controversial Experiment

One brave—or, many people later said, foolhardy—researcher tried to put corrective genes into human patients before these questions had been answered. He was Martin Cline, a specialist in blood diseases at the University of California at Los Angeles (UCLA).

In the United States and most other countries, new drugs or other medical treatments must go through a complicated series of steps before being tested on human beings. The scientists who develop the treatments must try them first on cells grown in the laboratory. If the treatments work in cells, they are then tested on small animals such as mice and, finally, on monkeys or other primates. Armed with results from all these tests, the researchers present proposals for human trials to a series of agencies. They begin with review boards at their own institutions and end, in the United States, with the federal Food and Drug Administration (FDA). Only after all these groups give their approval can human tests go ahead.

Cline developed a way to put a gene that coded for part of the human hemoglobin molecule into cells. Instead of putting the gene into altered whole viruses, he combined it with certain genes taken from viruses. He put this recombinant DNA into mice and showed that some of their blood cells became able to make the human protein. Then, in 1979, before the results of his mouse tests had been published, Cline asked UCLA's review board for permission to test the treatment on human beings with defective hemoglobin genes. Concerned about the safety of putting recombinant DNA into people, which had never been done before, the board rejected the proposal.

On July 10, 1980, Cline nonetheless gave his treatment to a patient—in Israel, not the United States. The patient, a woman, had a hemoglobin-defect disease called thalassemia. He repeated the treatment on a second thalassemia patient in Italy shortly afterward.

Cline's therapy seemed to neither help nor hurt his patients. The added genes probably never functioned in their bodies. Even so, both scientists and government authorities criticized Cline severely when they learned of his experiments later in the year. They claimed that he had made his tests overseas to avoid the strict rules in the United States. Cline denied this, saying he could not find enough thalassemia patients in America. Nonetheless, he was forbidden to do any more research on gene treatments. His premature experiment, furthermore, made many officials suspicious of the whole idea of gene therapy. As a result, the NIH established a special subcommittee within the RAC to review all future proposals for human gene therapy. This group, as well as the FDA, would have to give its approval before any tests on human patients could take place.

A Persistent Researcher

In spite of this setback, a few researchers refused to give up on gene therapy. One was a physician-scientist from Tulsa, Oklahoma, named William French Anderson. French, as he is known, had been interested in genes since he first heard of them in the summer of 1954, just before he started college. Even then he was sure that scientists and doctors would someday cure diseases by repairing or replacing defective genes—and that he would be one of those scientists. There "were . . . two things I was going to do with my life," Anderson said later. "I was going to be in the Olympics, and I was going to cure defective molecules."[6]

In the 1960s Anderson helped Marshall Nirenberg decipher parts of the genetic code. After 1975 his work at the NIH was devoted almost entirely to gene therapy—even though, technically, no such thing yet existed. He tried to improve methods for getting genes into cells, but he became so frustrated that for a while, during the early 1980s, he gave up and concentrated on a second interest, sports medicine. (This interest had allowed him, after a fashion, to achieve his goal of taking part in the Olympics: He had been the physician for the United States tae kwon do team at the 1976 games in Seoul, Korea. Anderson himself is an expert in this martial art.)

Nothing could keep Anderson away from gene therapy for long, however. In 1984 he heard about an

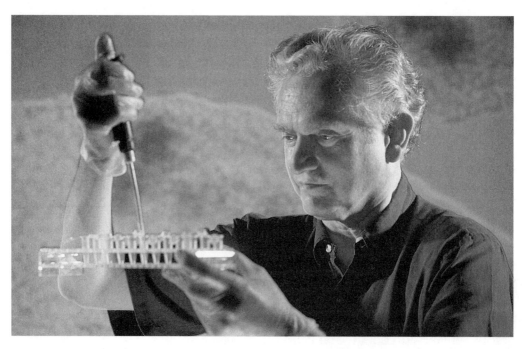

Marshall Nirenberg (pictured) deciphered parts of the genetic code in the 1960s with the help of French Anderson, who went on to develop the first successful human gene therapy.

inherited disease, ADA deficiency, that might be a candidate for such treatment. Children with this rare illness lack a working gene for an enzyme called adenosine deaminase (ADA). Certain cells in the body's defense system, the immune system, must have ADA in order to mature and remain healthy. Without it, the children's immune systems cannot function. Like people with AIDS, whose immune systems have been destroyed by a virus, these children come down with one infectious disease after another. Without treatment, most do not live to adulthood.

Gene therapy might work well for ADA deficiency, Anderson and a few other researchers realized, because the disease is caused by a mutation in a single gene that needs to be active only in certain blood cells. The gene in question had been identified in 1983. Anderson hoped that getting healthy ADA genes into even a small number of cells might give the children at least a minimal immune system. He found he shared this hope with Michael Blaese, another NIH scientist, who was a specialist in childhood immune diseases. The two men agreed to work together to develop gene therapy for ADA deficiency.

Planning a Treatment

As with all earlier attempts at gene therapy—and most later ones as well—putting new genes into enough cells to make a difference proved to be the hardest part of the job. Like most gene-therapy researchers at the time, Anderson's group planned to use a type of virus called a retrovirus to transfer the genes. Unlike other viruses, which merely insert their genes into a cell's nucleus, retroviruses can put theirs into the cell's own genome—its DNA. They are nature's own genetic engineers. Having a healthy gene placed in a cell's genome is useful to gene therapists because, at least in theory, it means that the added gene will be copied along with the cell's other genetic materal each time the cell reproduces. The gene will therefore continue to exist and function in all the cell's descendants. Other viruses cannot produce this result because their genes are not copied when cells reproduce.

There were two problems with retroviruses as gene "delivery trucks," however. One was safety. Many retroviruses produce deadly diseases such as AIDS and cancer. The viruses' disease-causing genes would be removed before they were used in gene therapy, but some researchers feared that the viruses might pick up copies of these genes from other viruses in the body and become dangerous again. Also, because retroviruses insert their genes randomly in the genome, there was a risk that they might produce cancer by damaging normal genes that control cell growth.

The other problem with retroviruses is that they can infect cells only when the cells are dividing. That means that many kinds of cells in the body are immune to them because these cells rarely or never divide. Unfortunately, stem cells, the blood-making cells in the bone marrow that Anderson wanted to infect, are among these. Anderson had little luck

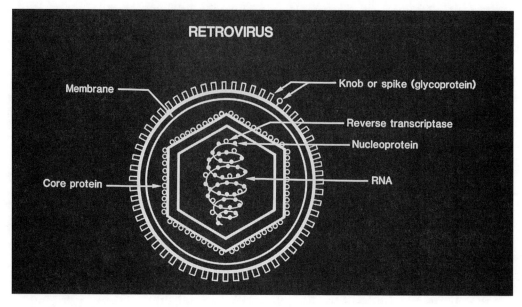

RETROVIRUS

Membrane

Knob or spike (glycoprotein)

Reverse transcriptase

Nucleoprotein

Core protein

RNA

Many retroviruses, parts of which are depicted by this illustration, carry deadly diseases.

transferring the ADA gene into mice, monkeys, or human stem cells in the laboratory.

Then Blaese had a brainstorm. The team should forget about stem cells, he said, and try putting the ADA gene into the few immune-system cells circulating in an ADA-deficient child's blood. These cells would not live as long as stem cells, so the treatment would have to be repeated, but it might be enough. A new member of the NIH team, thirty-six-year-old Iowa researcher Kenneth Culver, developed a technique for infecting these blood cells in the laboratory by the end of 1987. However, he still could not make the technique work in mice.

An Indirect Approach

Anderson had first asked the RAC's gene-therapy subcommittee for permission to test his therapy on ADA-deficient children in April 1987, while he was still trying to infect stem cells. The committee turned him down. Even after the NIH group explained Culver's new approach, the rejection continued. The group's lack of success in mice was one reason, and safety was another. Anderson explained that his team planned to remove immune-system cells from the children's blood, treat them with gene-carrying viruses in the laboratory, and reinject the cells rather than injecting viruses directly. Still, the subcommittee thought that putting foreign genes into humans was too risky.

A third reason for rejecting Anderson's therapy, in the committee's eyes, was that a much less controversial treatment for ADA deficiency had recently been invented. ADA, like most enzymes missing in inherited diseases, cannot simply be given as a pill because the stomach destroys protein. Even when injected, ADA breaks down quickly in the blood. In 1985, however, a Duke University scientist named Michael Hershfield had found that coating molecules of ADA with a substance called polyethylene glycol extended the enzyme's life in the blood. The resulting drug, PEG-ADA, did not cure ADA deficiency, but it gave children with the disease enough of an immune system to let them lead fairly normal lives. Anderson could promise no more for his gene therapy.

Anderson, Blaese, and Culver realized that they might have to take an indirect path to winning the committee's approval. Luckily for them, they found an ally in another NIH physician-researcher, Steven Rosenberg. At first Rosenberg, chief of surgery at the National Cancer Institute, was not working on gene therapy at all. He was trying to find ways to help the immune system fight cancer.

Rosenberg had discovered immune-system cells that seemed to head straight for tumors and attack the cancer cells within, leaving normal cells alone. In the mid-1980s he had taken blood or tumor tissue from dying cancer patients, stimulated the immune cells in it with a growth-inducing chemical, and then returned the cells to the patients' bodies. The treatment helped some people spectacularly but did nothing for others, and Rosenberg did not know why. To find out, he needed to learn where his special cells went after being reinjected and how long they survived.

When Rosenberg met Anderson and Blaese in March 1988, the researchers realized that they could help each other. For their part, Anderson and Blaese suggested to Rosenberg that he could use genetic engineering to track his cells. He could put a harmless gene into them from bacteria that made the bacteria resistant to a certain type of antibiotic. The gene could be added in the laboratory at the same time Rosenberg performed his other treatments on the cells. He could then reinject the treated cells. After they had been in the patients for a month or so, he could remove pieces of the patients' tumors and put them in laboratory dishes containing the antibiotic. Human cells do not normally make the resistance

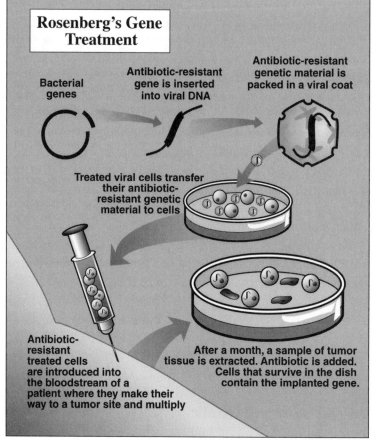

Rosenberg's Gene Treatment

Bacterial genes

Antibiotic-resistant gene is inserted into viral DNA

Antibiotic-resistant genetic material is packed in a viral coat

Treated viral cells transfer their antibiotic-resistant genetic material to cells

Antibiotic-resistant treated cells are introduced into the bloodstream of a patient where they make their way to a tumor site and multiply

After a month, a sample of tumor tissue is extracted. Antibiotic is added. Cells that survive in the dish contain the implanted gene.

Source: Eric S. Grace, *Biotechnology Unzipped*. Washington, D. C.: Joseph Henry Press, 1977.

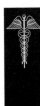

New Genes for Old

In giving gene therapy to children with ADA deficiency, French Anderson and the other scientists at the National Institutes of Health proposed to begin by snipping out genes that let retroviruses reproduce. In place of these genes, they would insert the human gene that codes for the ADA protein into the viruses' genomes.

Once they gained regulators' permission to begin human tests, the scientists would take blood from an ADA-deficient child. In their laboratory they would filter certain immune- system cells from the blood and mix the cells with the gene-carrying viruses. If all went well, the viruses would infect the cells and put their genetic material, including the normal ADA gene, into the cells' genomes. The researchers would then put the cells in a dish filled with nutrients and add a chemical that made cells multiply. After a week or so, they would reinject the cells into the child. They hoped that the cells with the new gene would begin making ADA in the child's body and produce enough of the vital substance to allow a healthy immune system to develop.

gene's protein, so any cells that survived in the dishes had to contain the implanted gene.

In turn, if Rosenberg could gain the RAC subcommittee's permission to do this marker-gene experiment and no problems resulted from it, the Anderson group's chances of getting approval for their ADA-deficiency tests would be greatly improved. Rosenberg seemed likely to have better success with the committee than Anderson's team for several reasons. First, his research centered on a disease that, unlike ADA deficiency, affects millions of people. Second, he would be treating only patients who were expected to die within a few months, so even a disastrous failure would not shorten their lives by much. And, finally, Rosenberg's treatment was not really gene therapy, since the inserted genes were not expected to either help or harm the patients.

A Giant Leap for Genetics

Committee members gave Rosenberg his own share of grilling, but both the RAC and the FDA finally granted him permission to go ahead. So it was that on May 22, 1989, as Rosenberg, Anderson, and Blaese watched anxiously, Maurice Kuntz, a fifty-two-year-old truck driver with advanced melanoma (a fast-growing, deadly skin cancer), received the first altered genes known to have survived in a human being. No problems occurred as the cells flowed into his body. ("I haven't grown a tail yet,"[7] Kuntz jokingly commented after a while.) Within a few hours, tests showed that cells containing the marker gene were circulating in his bloodstream. That day, echoing astronaut Neil Armstrong's famous words on first stepping onto the moon in 1969, Anderson put a sign on his office wall that read, "One small step for a gene, but a giant leap for genetics."[8]

As expected, the treatment had no lasting effect on Kuntz's cancer, and he died less than a year later. Nonetheless, Rosenberg and Anderson were encouraged. The genes seemed to make Kuntz no worse, and Rosenberg was able to detect his altered cells for several months. The group repeated the treatment on seven more dying cancer patients, with similar results.

Anderson and Blaese, meanwhile, went back to seeking permission for their ADA-deficiency therapy. They still got nowhere, however, until they heard about an Italian researcher named Claudio Bordignon. Bordignon was also designing a gene treatment for ADA deficiency—and, unlike the NIH group, he had made it work in mice that lacked immune systems. Blaese, who had met Bordignon at a scientific conference, begged him to tell the RAC subcommittee about his experiments because they provided the evidence of success in animals that the committee had been demanding. Even though Bordignon was, in a sense, the NIH group's competitor, he finally agreed to help his fellow scientists. Bordignon's testimony at a RAC meeting on July 30, 1990, "made a big difference in . . . how the subcommittee thought,"[9] Ken Culver said later.

The committee's last requirement was that children given the new therapy go on receiving PEG-ADA as well. This would make the effect of the therapy hard to judge, since any improvement in the children's condition might be due to either the gene treatment or the drug. However, the PEG-ADA would protect the children in case the gene therapy failed. Anderson's group agreed to the request.

Ashi Makes History

At the same July meeting, the NIH group told the committee about the child they had chosen to receive the first therapy. She was a solemn, dark-haired little girl named Ashanthi DeSilva—Ashi for short. Ashi's parents, Raj and Van DeSilva, had originally come from Sri Lanka, but they now lived in North Olmstead, a suburb of Cleveland, Ohio. Raj was a senior researcher in chemical engineering for the B. F. Goodrich Company. Ashi was a good choice for the gene treatment, Anderson and Blaese explained, because PEG-ADA did not seem to be helping her, but her body had not yet been severely damaged by infections. They said that if all went well with Ashi, they would also give the treatment to a second little girl, Cynthia (Cindy) Cutshall. "We had real examples . . . , and I think that was very important for the committee," Blaese later told Jeff Lyon and Peter Gorner. "It took it away from the abstract."[10]

At the end of the July meeting, the RAC voted twelve to one to let the Anderson-Blaese group go ahead with their treatment. By September the FDA gave its permission as well. On September 5, three days after Ashi's fourth birthday, Culver removed some of the little girl's blood and took it to the team's laboratory to begin the treatment. Then, on September 14, they put the immune-system cells with their new gene cargo back into Ashi's blood while she calmly watched television from her hospital bed. Anderson told reporters that the moment was not only a scientific triumph but "a cultural breakthrough, . . . an event that changes the way that we as a society think about ourselves."[11]

CHAPTER 3

Repairing Damaged Genes

By the year 2000 Ashanthi DeSilva had grown from a frail, serious-faced four-year-old into a smiling, active girl on the edge of adolescence. She had not had a gene treatment in seven years, though she had received eleven between September 1990 and August 1992. She still took PEG-ADA shots, but the dose was a mere quarter of the amount a child her age with the disease would need without gene therapy. Although only about a fourth of Ashi's immune cells produced ADA, this apparently was enough to give her body a basically normal defense system. She went to school, played basketball, and in general led an ordinary life. She was still, as French Anderson had described her in a 1995 article, "a healthy, vibrant [girl] who loves life and does *everything*."[12] Cindy Cutshall has done equally well.

Unfortunately, in spite of researchers' continuing efforts, few other children with inherited diseases have experienced Ashi DeSilva's happy ending. Both the public and many scientists believed that genetic cures for such diseases would start appearing within a few years of Ashi's groundbreaking treatment, but they were wrong. "We got a rude awakening," Anderson told an interviewer in 1999. "It is much more difficult to get genes into cells than we thought it would be, and once in the cells, genes were turned off after a few days or weeks."[13]

The Ideal Delivery Truck

In all kinds of gene therapy, the biggest problem has proved to be finding the right tools to get the genes into cells. Michael Blaese quotes a common saying in the field that "the three problems [with] gene therapy have been delivery, delivery, and delivery."[14] Another leading gene researcher, Inder Verma of the Salk Institute in La Jolla, California, says that the ideal gene carrier, or vector, would be "easy to make, . . . delivers genes at very high efficiency, . . . can infect a nondividing cell and . . . enables its therapeutic gene to become part and parcel of the chromosome."[15] A good vector also needs to be big enough to hold fairly large genes. It should be harmless to the body, and, finally, it should produce no reaction from the immune system. Unfortunately, no vector yet discovered or invented has all these characteristics.

Most of the gene-therapy vectors tested so far have been viruses. Each type has advantages and disadvantages. Retroviruses, which were used in most of the first gene-therapy experiments, can put genes directly into a cell's genome. This increases the chance that the genes will make their proteins permanently. The viruses cause little immune reaction and can hold large genes. However, as Anderson's group learned, retroviruses infect only rapidly dividing cells. Cells given genes by retroviruses also sometimes stop producing their new proteins after a few weeks. Finally, although no retrovirus used in gene therapy has yet been shown to harm a patient, a risk remains that the viruses will insert their genes in a way that causes cancer or some other kind of genome damage.

Dissatisfied with the results from retroviruses, many researchers in the mid-1990s began using a

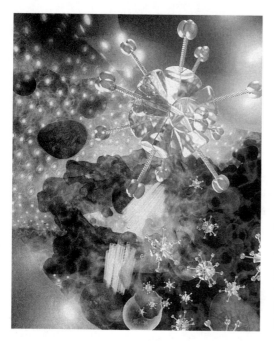

These capsules, made from adenoviruses, use a virus's natural infective ability to deliver genes into cells.

different virus as a gene vector. This virus, the adenovirus, is all too familiar to most people (whether they know its name or not) as one of the kinds of virus that cause colds. Adenoviruses easily infect nondividing as well as dividing cells, especially cells in the nose and lungs. They insert their genes easily into cell nuclei, although, unlike retroviruses, they do not put them in the genome. Adenoviruses are easy to grow in quantity and, being fairly large viruses, they can carry large genes. They can be engineered to seek out particular kinds of cells.

Clogged Lungs

Scientists felt that these features made adenoviruses an ideal choice for gene therapy to treat an inherited disease called cystic fibrosis. Cystic fibrosis is the most common fatal inherited disease in the United States, striking one out of about every three thousand children. The gene that causes it, which was identified in 1989, affects the way salt and water are pumped in and out of cells.

This defective gene creates problems in several parts of the body, including the digestive system, but its most severe effects are in the lungs. It makes thick mucus build up there and also blocks the effects of an antibiotic that certain lung cells make. As a result, bacteria can easily invade the lungs of cystic fibrosis patients, and these people suffer one chest infection after another. Antibiotics and other treatments now keep many people with cystic fibrosis alive until their twenties or thirties, but they must receive constant medical attention and cannot be cured. Gene therapy would be a real blessing to them.

Two teams of scientists corrected the cystic fibrosis gene defect in laboratory cells as early as 1990. Tests on mice and monkeys followed, and tests on humans began in 1993. In the cystic fibrosis treatments, unlike the ones given to Ashi DeSilva, gene-carrying viruses were put directly into the patients' bodies. This was the first time such a thing had been done in humans. In some versions of these early experiments, researchers dripped or sprayed liquid containing altered adenoviruses into patients' noses. In others, they put virus-containing liquid into the patients' lungs through a hollow tube called a bronchoscope.

The researchers had modified the adenoviruses so that they could not cause colds. Unfortunately, the patients' immune systems did not "realize" that the viruses were harmless. Immune cells attacked the invaders vigorously and destroyed most of them before they could deposit their gene cargo. As a result, signs of corrected gene activity appeared in only about 10 percent of the lung cells exposed to the virus,

Stages of Human Testing

Tests of gene therapy or any other new medical treatment on human beings take place in three stages.

Phase I tests: The treatment is given in different doses to small numbers of patients, often ones who have not been helped by other treatments. The main purpose of this test is to find out what doses of the treatment are safe and what problems (if any) it causes.

Phase II tests: The best doses of the treatment are given to somewhat larger numbers of people. This test continues to check safety, but it also helps researchers find out how effective the treatment is.

Phase III tests: The treatment is given to larger numbers of patients, perhaps several hundred. Some patients receive the new treatment, while others receive the standard treatment for their disease. Often neither the patients nor their doctors are told which treatment they are receiving. This is done because people sometimes feel better simply because they know they are getting an exciting new treatment. This test lets scientists compare the new treatment with existing ones.

Patients in all tests are told about the treatment and any known or suspected harm that it may cause. They (or their parents, if they are minors) must sign a form saying that they have been informed about the treatment and agree, or consent, to receiving it during the test.

and the activity did not last long. Worse still, the immune reaction became stronger each time the viruses were introduced. This was a problem because the scientists expected to have to give the treatment many times to each patient. The immune attack sometimes destroyed normal as well as virus-infected lung cells, making some patients sicker, at least temporarily.

Ducking the Immune System

Researchers have been exploring ways to overcome the problems revealed in these early tests. Some experimenters have removed more genes from the adenoviruses in the hope that this will make the viruses seem less threatening to the immune system. Others have suggested giving the adenovirus treatment to fetuses, or unborn babies, that have been shown to carry the defective gene. The immune system is much less active before birth than it is afterward, so a fetus's system probably would not react to the viruses. This treatment has been effective in mice, but neither it nor any other gene therapy has yet been tried on human fetuses.

Some scientists think the best way to avoid immune reactions is to transfer genes without using viruses. They have experimented with putting genes into microscopic blobs of fat called liposomes. Liposomes insert themselves into cell membranes, which are made partly of similar material, and release their contents inside the cells. The immune system does not react to liposomes, and the oily spheres are completely harmless and

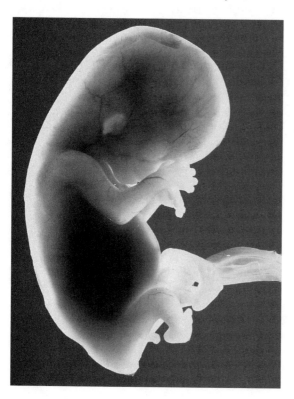

Scientists have suggested giving adenovirus treatment to fetuses that carry defective genes.

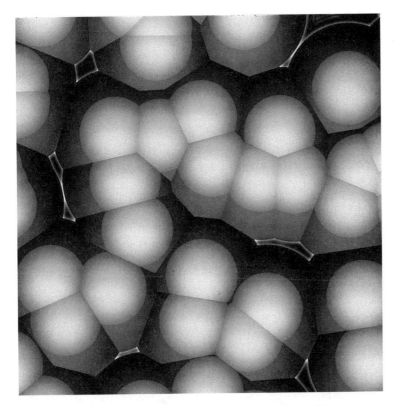

Microscopic spheres of fat called liposomes can insert themselves into cell membranes, releasing their contents inside the cells.

fairly easy to manufacture. So far, however, liposomes have not proved nearly as effective at putting genes into cells as viruses are. Even when the DNA they carry does enter cells, the cells usually destroy it before it can reach the nucleus or make protein.

Other researchers are trying out different viruses as vectors, because the immune system does not attack all viruses as vigorously as it does adenoviruses. Some of the best results so far have come from a virus called an adeno-associated virus. Unlike adenoviruses, adeno-associated viruses can slip past the immune system's sentries like stealthy ninjas. As far as is known, they cause no disease in humans. They infect nondividing as well as dividing cells, and they insert their genes into the genome, leading to long-lasting effects. The main problem with adeno-associated viruses as gene carriers is that they are fairly small, as viruses go. This means that there

is room for only small genes in the "hollowed-out"
space left after the genes that let the viruses reproduce have been removed.

Treating the "Royal Disease"

Adeno-associated viruses have been tested as carriers
in gene therapy for cystic fibrosis. They have also produced promising results in gene therapy for one form
of hemophilia, the "royal disease" that affected the
Russian prince Alexis. Normal blood clotting depends
on a number of proteins, including two called factor
VIII and factor IX. People with the more common type
of hemophilia, hemophilia A, lack the gene that makes
factor VIII. About 13,500 people in the United States,
almost all males, have this form of the disease.
Another 5,000 or so instead lack the gene for factor IX
and are said to have hemophilia B. In both forms of
hemophilia, internal bleeding damages joints as well as
causing other problems. "My knees don't bend. I walk
with a cane, sort of stiff-legged, like Frankenstein [the
monster],"[16] says Mark Ross, a hemophiliac in his late
thirties.

To control joint damage and dangerous bouts of
bleeding, people with hemophilia must have frequent transfusions of whole blood or injections of
purified clotting factors. These treatments have carried their own dangers. Until recent years hemophiliacs ran a high risk of being infected with viruses
carried in blood, such as those that cause AIDS or
hepatitis (a serious liver disease). That risk is much
smaller today, both because tests can identify viruses
in blood before it is used and because genetically
engineered bacteria can be used to make the clotting
factors. These recombinant factors are very expensive, however. They can cost hemophiliacs and their
families more than $100,000 a year.

A number of scientists think hemophilia is a good
choice for gene therapy for several reasons. The genes
that cause both forms of the disease are well known.

As with ADA deficiency, even a small quantity of the missing protein—as little as 5 percent of the normal amount—would help people with the disease considerably. This means that the treatment might still work even if only small numbers of blood-producing cells were infected. Production of larger amounts of the factors would do no harm, however. This is important because the amount of protein that added genes produce is hard to control. Finally, a simple blood test can show whether a treatment is working.

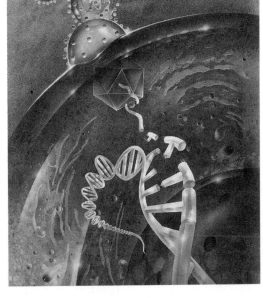

This illustration shows how gene therapy introduces new, beneficial genes to cells through a viral messenger.

Big and Little Genes

In mid-1999 Katherine High at Children's Hospital in Philadelphia and Mark Kay of the Stanford University School of Medicine began giving several hemophilia-B patients muscle injections of adeno-associated viruses carrying the gene for factor IX. Avigen, a biotechnology company in Alameda, California, helped to prepare the gene treatment. None of the patients showed any side effects (unwanted or harmful effects) from the therapy. Furthermore, within two months two of the three were making detectable factor IX. They produced only about 1 percent of the amount normal people make, but that was enough to reduce the size and number of the factor IX injections they had to have.

The new genes were still working nine months later, but not as powerfully. This may mean that the treatment would have to be given many times. As researchers found out when testing treatments for cystic fibrosis, the immune system reacts more strongly when "invasions" are repeated. Some people with hemophilia even fear that gene therapy might make them become allergic to the injected blood factors they must now take. That would leave them with no treatment options at all. In spite of these concerns, tests of the new therapy continue.

Gene treatments for hemophilia B have proved easier to design than those for hemophilia A because the gene that codes for factor VIII is much larger than the one that codes for factor IX. It will not fit inside adeno-associated viruses. Some researchers are falling back on larger viruses to ferry this monster gene. In 1999, for instance, Inder Verma and his coworkers at the Salk Institute were doing animal tests using a "tamed" version of perhaps the most feared retrovirus of all—HIV (human immunodeficiency virus), the virus that causes AIDS. Obviously, many safety tests would have to take place before this virus would be given to humans, if it ever is. Nonetheless, Verma thinks that HIV and related retroviruses, a group called lentiviruses, eventually will make very good vectors for gene therapy. Unlike other retroviruses, they can infect cells that are not dividing. They can hold large genes, and they are experts at avoiding the immune system.

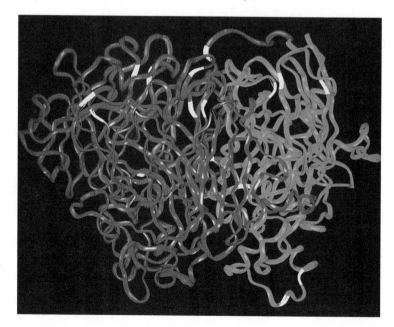

Pictured is a computer-generated model of the gene that codes for factor VIII protein.

Other researchers, such as David Roth of Beth Israel Deaconess Medical Center in Boston, are working around the gene-size problem by skipping viruses entirely. Instead, they are using a technique called electroporation to put factor VIII genes into skin cells taken from people with hemophilia. In the laboratory an electric current temporarily opens the cells' membranes and lets the foreign DNA enter. Surgeons then transplant the treated cells into the fat just under the skin of the patients' abdomens. Roth and his coworkers reported in December 2000 that the blood of four out of six patients given this treatment clotted faster than it had before, though it was still far from normal. If this treatment works dependably, it would avoid the risk of illness caused by either viruses or immune reactions to them. Some scientists question, however, whether enough cells will take up and keep the gene.

Strengthening Weak Muscles

Researchers have also had some luck in using gene therapy to treat another life-threatening inherited disease, muscular dystrophy. Muscular dystrophy is actually a group of diseases, each of which is caused by a mutation in a different gene. All cause muscles to break down, becoming weaker and more useless. Most children with these diseases do not survive into adulthood. The most common form, Duchenne muscular dystrophy, is caused by a defect in the gene that makes a protein called dystrophin. This sex-linked disease affects about twenty thousand boys in the United States, one child in every thirty-five hundred births. It is one of the most common inherited diseases caused by a defect in a single gene.

The dystrophin gene was identified in 1986. Unfortunately, this gene, like the gene for factor VIII, is too big to fit into most virus carriers. Xiao Xiao and other researchers at the University of Pittsburgh School of Medicine are trying to work around this problem by breaking the gene into two parts. They put each part into a different group of adeno-associated viruses. The parts apparently rejoin inside cells, producing a working dystrophin gene.

Xiao's group has also done animal tests on miniaturized forms of the dystrophin gene that contain just its most important sequences. These tests also used adeno-associated viruses, which were injected into the muscles of mice with a disease very similar to Duchenne dystrophy. Up to 90 percent of the fibers in the treated muscles began to make dystrophin, the researchers announced in November 2000. Better still, they were still making it a year later. The treated muscles were "indistinguishable from healthy muscle,"[17] Xiao said.

Scientists have had even better luck treating a type called limb-girdle muscular dystrophy, which chiefly affects the muscles of the upper arms and legs. This disease is rarer than Duchenne dystrophy. Like hemophilia B, however, it has proven easier to treat than the more common form of the disease because the defective genes that cause it are smaller. Limb-girdle dystrophy is caused by mutations in any of the four genes that make proteins in a group called the sarcoglycan complex. The membranes of muscle cells must have all these proteins in order to work properly. Each sarcoglycan gene is small enough to fit into an adeno-associated virus.

Besides trying to create gene therapy for Duchenne dystrophy, Xiao's research group at the University of Pittsburgh is working on a treatment for limb-girdle dystrophy. In October 1999 Xiao announced that he had injected adeno-associated viruses carrying sarcoglycan genes into the leg muscles of hamsters that had a disease like limb-girdle dystrophy. They tested the treated muscles after a month. The muscles, Xiao said, had returned to normal size and increased nearly 100 percent in strength. At about the same time, researchers at the University of Pennsylvania's Institute for Human Gene Therapy were planning to test a similar treatment in foot muscles of human patients.

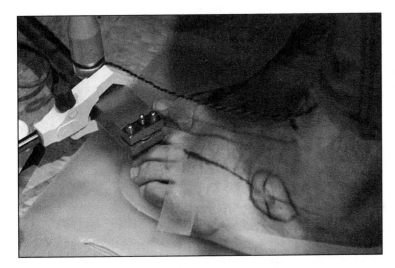

A patient suffering from limb-girdle muscular dystrophy of the foot prepares for his first gene therapy injection.

The First Genetic Cure?

Perhaps the most encouraging news in tests of gene therapy for inherited diseases so far came in April 2000. Marina Cavazzana-Calvo and other researchers at the Necker Hospital in Paris announced that they had successfully treated two babies with an immune-system disease. This disease, X-linked severe combined immunodeficiency disease (SCID), has effects much like those of ADA deficiency, though it is caused by a different defective gene. It afflicts about one child in every fifty thousand births. X-linked SCID affects only boys because the recessive gene that causes it, like the one that causes hemophilia, is carried on the X chromosome. This gene codes for a protein that lets immune-system cells respond to certain chemicals that make them multiply. This protein, like ADA, is necessary for the immune system to function.

The French researchers gave gene treatments to the babies when they were a little less than a year old. The therapy was somewhat like that given to Ashi DeSilva, except that this time the scientists used cells from bone marrow rather than from blood. In the ten years since Ashi's treatment, it has become much easier to obtain stem cells, the long-lived blood-making cells, from marrow and make them multiply in the laboratory. The scientists removed a small amount of marrow from the babies and, in the laboratory, combined it with gene-carrying retroviruses and a mixture of substances that encouraged the cells to take up the genes. (This "cocktail is at the heart of the breakthrough,"[18] an article in *Business Week* claimed.) They reinjected the cells three days later.

Three months after the treatment, tests showed that the babies' immune systems were beginning to develop normally. Until then the babies had been kept in a special hospital nursery, protected from germs, and visited only by people wearing sterile masks and gowns. After the successful tests, however, they were allowed to go home and live like normal children. Their immune systems were still functioning well ten months after the treatment, the researchers said. If their immune systems continue to work properly, these babies may become the first people ever judged to be cured of a disease by gene therapy.

Challenges for Gene Therapy

Many genes that cause inherited diseases were identified in the 1990s. Furthermore, in June 2000 government and private scientists announced that the Human Genome Project, which was to determine the base sequence of the entire collection of genes in a human being, had been completed. Scientists still will need years of work to discover what individual genes this listing contains and what those genes do. Their efforts are sure to reveal numerous new targets for gene therapy.

Several problems must be solved before gene therapy can treat even the simplest inherited diseases successfully, however. Improving the safety and effectiveness of viruses and other vectors is still the biggest one. Getting the vectors to put their genes into the right cells is also difficult. Often scientists want a gene to work only in certain types of cells, such as cancer cells, blood cells, or lung cells. Some

The Bubble Boy

In The New Healers: The Promise and Problems of Molecular Medicine in the Twenty-First Century, *William R. Clark describes the most famous victim of X-linked SCID.*

The nation became suddenly aware of SCID through the dramatic and ultimately tragic case of a young boy named David, who was born in Texas in 1971. (David's full name was never made public.) . . .

[David's doctors] hope[d] that if he could be kept alive long enough in the absence of disease, his immune system might somehow "kick in." . . . [As a baby he was kept in a sterile, or germ-free, incubator.] When he began to crawl and eventually to stand, he was moved into a sterile tent that allowed some freedom of movement. . . . The tent eventually . . . [was expanded into] "the Bubble," an ingenious complex of interconnecting plastic tubes that allowed him to move around and explore, in an environment full of variously shaped and colored objects to stimulate . . . vision and touch. It was constructed in such a way as to allow maximal interactivity with family and playmates on the outside. . . . His nurses and tutors found him to be a bright, somewhat mischievous youngster. . . .

But his immune system never developed. As David continued to grow, it became clear that something had to be done. . . . What if he tried to break out of his bubble? . . .

Finally, it was decided to give David a bone marrow transplant, with his fifteen-year-old sister Katherine as the donor [in the hope that the marrow could make immune-system cells for him]. . . . Everything seemed to go well at first. But a few weeks later he developed . . . signs of a viral infection. David's condition grew rapidly worse; he finally died [124 days after the] . . . transplant. He was twelve years old.

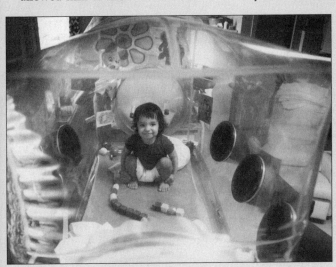

Young David plays in his plastic bubble.

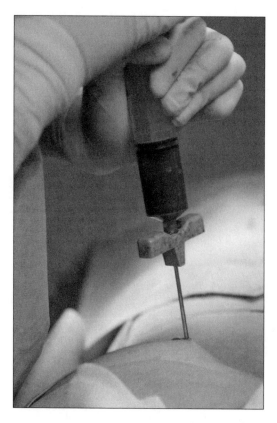

A physician removes a small amount of bone marrow that will be mixed with gene-carrying retroviruses.

genes might be harmful if they are active in the wrong cells. Even when this is not the case, infecting every cell in the body is impractical, so researchers want to focus their efforts on the types of cells where the gene will do the most good. Some researchers are modifying the protein shells of viruses so that the viruses will be attracted to particular types of cells.

Timing is important in gene therapy, too. Many genes are active only at certain times in the life of a cell or a living thing. In some cases, the body would be harmed if a gene were "turned on" all the time or at the wrong time. To control the timing of genes, some researchers have put DNA sequences called promoters into virus carriers along with genes. The promoters tell the genes when to turn on. Others engineer genes so that the genes become active only when stimulated by a drug. James Wilson, director of the Institute for Human Gene Therapy at the University of Pennsylvania, says that in the future, triggers like this "will be . . . a genetic rheostat [a device used to dim or brighten lights]. The gene will not work until you take a pill, and the more pills you take, the more the gene will be expressed—and if you want to cut off the supply [of gene product], you simply stop taking the pill."[19]

Besides these scientific problems, gene therapy for most inherited diseases also faces the challenge of economics. Developing a new drug or other medical treatment is a tremendously expensive and time-consuming process, often requiring at least ten years and millions of dollars. Most drug and biotechnology companies want to make this effort only for diseases common enough to ensure that many customers will want the finished product. Most inherited diseases do not meet this requirement. Inherited diseases caused by a mutation in a single gene—the most obvious candidates for gene therapy—account for just 2 percent of all diseases.

Of 409 proposals for human gene-therapy trials submitted to the National Institutes of Health by December 2000, only 50 were for inherited diseases. Research on these diseases continues, however. Scientists pursue gene therapy for inherited diseases not only for humanitarian reasons but because techniques that they learn in attempting to treat these relatively simple illnesses can be applied to gene therapy for conditions with more complex genetics as well. These include major killers such as cancer, heart disease, and AIDS.

CHAPTER 4

Treating Commom Killers

When people in the future think of gene therapy, they probably will not think of someone like Ashi DeSilva, a child stricken with a rare inherited disease. Instead, they may picture a person like Floyd Stokes. Genes did not cause Stokes's health problem, at least not in as direct a way as they caused Ashi's. Still, genes may cure him.

Feeding Starved Hearts

Stokes is a peanut farmer in Texas. In the late 1990s, like almost 12.5 million other people in the United States, he had a heart that was starved for oxygen. Fatty deposits had blocked most of his coronary arteries, which carry the blood that nourishes his heart. As a result, he had had several heart attacks. He felt exhausted and suffered chest pain, or angina, every time he did the slightest exercise. He could hardly even walk around his house.

Doctors commonly use several treatments to help people like Stokes. One is angioplasty, in which a tiny balloon is moved through a blood vessel until the blocked part is reached, then inflated to push the walls of the vessel apart. A tubelike device called a stent is then inserted to keep the vessel open. Another is a bypass operation, in which surgeons use a healthy vein from another part of the body to replace the blocked artery. Each year about 500,000 people in the United States have angioplasties, and another 400,000 have bypass operations.

Unfortunately, fairly often the newly opened or transplanted vessels become blocked again after a few months or years. Some people have to have surgery several times. Eventually their hearts are so damaged that the surgery will no longer work. Floyd Stokes, along with almost a quarter of a million other Americans, had reached that point.

On May 26, 1998, Stokes became one of sixteen patients to receive experimental gene therapy from Jeffrey Isner, a professor of medicine and pathology at Tufts University School of Medicine in Boston. Isner's treatment is designed to help people's own bodies grow the blood vessels their hearts need. At St. Elizabeth's Medical Center, he injected Stokes's heart with a gene that makes a protein called vascular endothelial growth factor, or VEGF, one of a group of natural substances called growth factors. Douglas W. Losordo, a member of Isner's team, later explained the advantage of this kind of therapy over the usual treatments for blocked vessels:

Gene therapy may someday be used to replace arteries choked by fatty deposits like those pictured here.

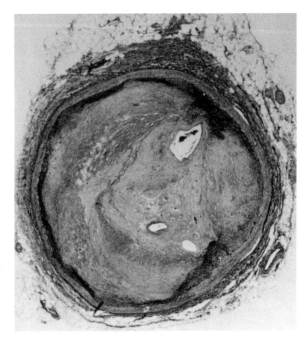

> Gene therapy is attractive because we are capitalizing on a natural process already in place in the body and trying to augment [add to] that system temporarily in order to sort of kick-start a process that we know can alleviate [relieve] symptoms and improve blood

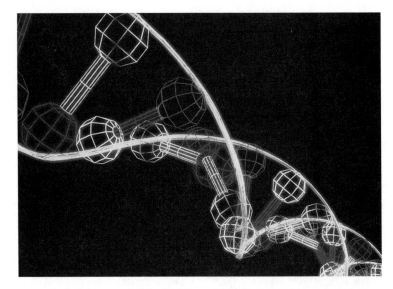

A computer representation of a segment of DNA. Rather than depending on virus carriers, Jeffrey Isner used "naked DNA" made from genetically engineered bacteria.

flow. Unlike a lot of pharmacological [drug] therapies in which a totally foreign substance is put into the body to help it, there is really nothing particularly foreign being introduced here.[20]

Unlike many other gene-therapy researchers, Isner used "naked DNA" rather than depending on virus carriers. Such DNA, made from genetically engineered bacteria, causes little immune response. It also cannot damage cell DNA as viruses sometimes can. Many experimenters have had trouble getting large numbers of cells to take up naked DNA, and genes introduced in this way may not function for long. However, the success of Isner's experiments so far suggests that brief expression in a fairly small number of cells may be enough. Imitating the Marine Corps slogan, Isner says, "All we're looking for are a few good genes."[21]

Back at Work

Stokes was not Isner's first patient. People can suffer blockages in the arteries in their legs as well as their hearts, sometimes resulting in damage so severe that the legs must be amputated. Beginning in 1994 after successful animal experiments, Isner tested his therapy first in people with blocked leg arteries. He treated ten legs in nine patients, giving each person two injections of VEGF DNA in their leg muscles four weeks apart. He reported in 1996 that blood flow had improved in eight of the ten treated legs. In most cases, he said, the improvement was as great as that seen with successful bypass surgery or angioplasty.

In 1998 Isner began testing the VEGF treatments on a small number of people who, like Stokes, had severe heart disease. All had had heart bypass surgeries, angioplasties, or both but could no longer have surgery. The results of this phase I study were encouraging—some would say spectacular. Measurements confirmed that the blood flow in all the patients' hearts had increased. The patients had been taking the drug nitroglycerin each time they had a bout of chest pain, consuming an average of sixty pills a week. Among eleven patients followed up for more than ninety days, the average nitroglycerin use dropped to 2.5 pills a week. Six, including Stokes, said they no longer had any angina at all.

Less than a year after the treatment, Stokes was back at work on his farm. "I ride horses and I run tractors," he said in early 1999. "You have to be in pretty good shape to do what I do."[22] His wife, Jean, stated, "Our life is now filled with hope."[23]

Isner said early in 2000 that his group had treated about seventy-two patients with the new therapy in two phase I studies and that "most of them—approximately 90 percent—have done exceptionally well."[24] He had kept track of a few patients for up to two years and found no signs that they needed further gene treatments. He reported good results from a later study in August 2000 as well. "There has been great concern about whether gene therapy works. This is very solid evidence that it does,"[25] Isner told reporters. He said that even some areas of heart muscle that had appeared to be dead were revived by the treatment.

If these treatments continue to be successful, they may make angioplasty or bypass surgery unnecessary for some people. It may even become possible to prevent heart attacks by inserting blood vessel genes into heart muscle along with a promoter that becomes active only if oxygen concentrations in the muscle drop to dangerously low levels.

Questions remain to be answered about Isner's gene therapy before it (or any of the similar approaches to treating heart disease that other research groups are testing) becomes widely available, however. Perhaps the chief one is whether the treatment might accidentally spur the growth of cancer. Tumors need new blood vessels just as much as blocked hearts do, and they make substances much like VEGF to stimulate blood vessel growth. Disturbingly, one of Isner's heart patients had a cancer that tripled in size soon after the gene treatment.

Isner's program is typical of gene-therapy research today. Although gene therapy was first proposed as a way to treat inherited diseases, most therapies being tested now are aimed at illnesses such as heart disease, cancer, and AIDS, which affect far greater numbers of people. Designing gene therapy for such diseases is much harder than doing so for single-gene problems such as ADA deficiency because the illnesses involve defects in multiple genes, many of which have not been identified. Gene therapy, therefore, has had to move beyond replacing damaged genes. Isner's therapy, for instance, uses VEGF genes not to replace a missing or damaged gene for this growth factor, but rather to help his patients' bodies repair the damage produced by other causes.

Gene Therapy for Cancer

Gene therapists have paid more attention to cancer than to any other single disease. Of 409 proposed human tests of gene therapy submitted to the NIH for review by the end of 2000, 249 were for cancer treatments. Gene therapy has seemed a natural choice for cancer because, beginning in the 1970s, scientists had

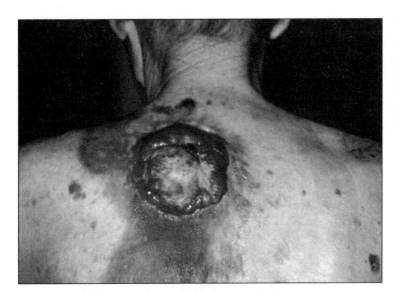

Tumors, like this skin cancer, are caused by genetic defects. Gene therapy researchers have devoted much effort to developing treatments for cancer.

learned that all cancers are due to mutations in genes that directly or indirectly affect cells' life span and power to reproduce. These defects cause the cells to live longer and reproduce much more often than is normal for their type. Eventually the cells grow into masses called tumors.

The genetic defects that cause cancer are inherited in only about 1 percent of cases. The rest are mutations that occur in individual cells during a person's lifetime. The mutations may happen by chance, or they may result from damage by factors in the environment such as chemicals in cigarette smoke or ultraviolet radiation in sunlight. In some cases, the mutated gene, called an oncogene (cancer gene), speeds up cell growth directly. In others, a mutation inactivates a type of gene called a tumor suppressor gene, whose normal job is to put a brake on cell growth. Usually, several different genes within a cell must be damaged before the cell becomes cancerous. The damage often accumulates over many years, which is why cancer is most common among older people.

The fact that cancer involves multiple genes—and different genes in different types of cancer and different people—has made developing gene therapy for this disease difficult. It probably also means that there will never be a single type of gene therapy that can stop all cancers. However, researchers in the late 1990s developed and began testing several promising gene therapies aimed at particular cancers.

A Killer Gene

One of the most creative gene therapies for cancer got its start as a backup safety measure for the treatment given to Ashanthi DeSilva. Michael Blaese and Kenneth Culver worried that the retroviruses they were using might accidentally insert an ADA gene at a spot in the genome of one of Ashi's blood cells that would activate an oncogene or turn off a tumor suppressor gene. "We wanted to build a self-destruct mechanism into these viruses," Blaese recalled in 1998. "If the worst happened—if cancer occurred— we could pull the plug and kill the cells."[26]

The researchers decided to give the cells not only the ADA gene but a second gene taken from a different family of viruses, the herpesviruses. (The most common kind of herpesvirus causes small sores on the lip called cold sores.) This gene makes herpesviruses very sensitive to an antiviral drug called gancyclovir. Normal human cells lack the herpes gene, so the drug does not harm them. If Ashi developed cancer as a result of her therapy, the theory went, the researchers would simply give her gancyclovir and it would destroy the rogue cells.

Blaese and Culver soon realized that their proposed therapy might help far more people than Ashi. "Instead of using it as a fail-safe device, we could kill cancer with it,"[27] Blaese says. They hoped to infect the rapidly dividing cells in cancerous tumors with a retrovirus carrying the herpes gene, then give the cancer patients gancyclovir to kill the cells.

As a first test, Blaese and Culver used a retrovirus to put the herpes gene into laboratory cells and showed that gancyclovir could then kill the cells. As usual, the

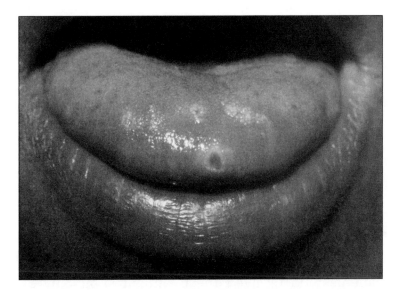

Small sores on a person's tongue or lips, called cold sores, are the result of herpes simplex I virus.

retroviruses infected only dividing cells. This suggested that the treatment would not harm noncancerous cells because those cells would not be dividing and therefore would not receive the gene.

The scientists were even more pleased when they tried their treatment on animals with cancer. Although only a fairly small percentage of cancer cells apparently took up the herpes gene, Blaese and Culver found that the gancyclovir killed cancer cells near those with the gene as well as the cells actually containing it. They were not sure why this "bystander effect" occurred, but they were glad it did because it made the treatment much more effective than it otherwise would have been.

Attacking Brain Cancer

The two researchers decided to try their new treatment on a kind of brain tumor called glioblastoma. This cancer, which affects some ten thousand people in the United States each year, is the most common as well as the deadliest type of brain cancer. It kills most of its victims within a year. It is very hard to halt with standard cancer treatments—surgery, radiation, and chemotherapy (drug treatment)—because it grows and spreads quickly. It does not travel outside the brain, however, which means that only cells in and near the existing tumors would need to be infected. Normal brain cells do not usually divide, so they would not be expected to take up the herpes gene. Blaese and Culver tested the treatment on mice with glioblastomas and showed that it completely destroyed the tumors without harming the animals.

The first human test of the new therapy, called GLI-328, took place in 1992. The scientists tried the treatment on a small number of patients with advanced glioblastoma that had not responded to standard treatments. For such an early stage of testing, the results were encouraging. Tumors in four of the ten patients who received the treatment shrank by as much as half, although all the cancers eventually grew back and killed the patients. In a second test with an improved virus vector and more patients, conducted in 1995 and 1996, six of the thirty-one people tested were still alive four years later. "We've never seen anything like it with any other therapy,"[28] said Mitchel Burger of the University of California at San Francisco, where the test occurred.

A phase III test, involving about 250 patients in forty cancer centers around the world, began in the

A Revolutionary Treatment

The experimental treatment that Michael Blaese and Kenneth Culver developed for glioblastoma begins with a surgeon opening the skull of a person with this deadly brain cancer. Guided by three-dimensional maps of the brain prepared earlier by computer imaging, the surgeon removes as much of the tumor as possible. The surgeon then injects viruses carrying a herpes virus gene into multiple spots around the area where the tumor was removed.

Two weeks pass. During this time, the researchers hope, the viruses will insert the herpes genes into any glioblastoma cells remaining in the patient's brain. At the end of the two-week period, the patient begins receiving injections of gancyclovir twice a day. This treatment continues for another two weeks. The researchers expect that the cancer cells containing the added herpes gene will convert the drug into a substance that kills them and any other cancer cells that are nearby.

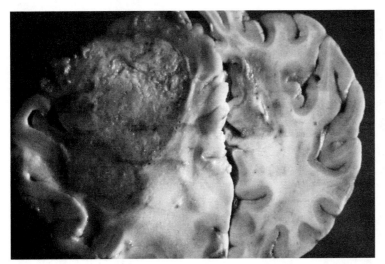

This cross section of the brain shows cancerous brain tissue. The type of brain cancer called glioblastoma is often lethal because it grows and spreads quickly.

late 1990s. Unfortunately, the results of this test were disappointing. Overall, the gene therapy did not help patients live any longer than surgery and radiation alone. The chief problem seemed to be that not as many cancer cells took up functioning herpes genes as the researchers had hoped. Scientists are now trying to find more effective genes and viruses to use. They also hope to increase the number of cancer cells killed by the "bystander effect." This treatment is still considered very promising, but, as with other gene therapies, it is likely to need years of refinement before it becomes a standard part of medicine—if it ever does. Several other types of gene therapy for glioblastoma are also being tested.

Guardian of the Genome

Other experimental gene therapies for cancer focus on a tumor suppressor gene called p53, which is damaged in almost half of all cancers. This gene, which some scientists have called the guardian of the genome, makes a cell destroy itself when the gene detects signs of abnormal cell division or DNA damage that cannot be repaired. In cells where this important gene no longer functions, reproduction can speed along like a car with no brakes.

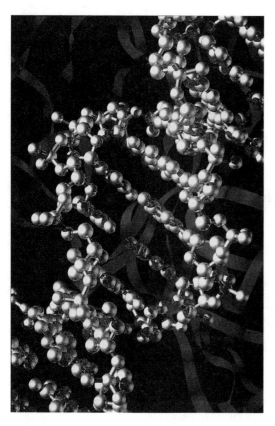

Called guardian of the genome, the tumor suppressor gene p53 (pictured in a model of DNA) makes a cell destroy itself when the gene detects signs of abnormality.

Jack Roth and his coworkers at the M. D. Anderson Cancer Center in Houston, Texas, have used adenoviruses to put healthy copies of the p53 gene into lung cancer cells. When they tried the treatment on animals, Roth told a *Texas Monthly* interviewer in 1998, it "not only corrected the p53 defect but . . . also caused the cancer cells to self-destruct. I was astonished to see that. Cancer cells have all these different genetic deletions [missing parts] and defects, and here we were correcting just one and having this profound effect."[29]

The p53 therapy was tested on humans with lung cancer beginning in 1994. Like the glioblastoma treatment, it made some of the patients' tumors shrink temporarily, but all of them grew back. Still, in the most recent experiments, which Roth described in 1999, the rate of cell "suicide" in the patients' tumors was at least twice what it had been before the therapy. Roth's and other groups are continuing to refine the treatment and to test it against other kinds of cancer.

Meanwhile, another research group, headed by Frank McCormick at ONYX Pharmaceuticals, a biotechnology company in Richmond, California, is taking an exactly opposite approach to p53. Instead of using adenoviruses to add the missing p53, they have altered these viruses to make them able to infect only cells in which the p53 gene is missing. Unlike the usual case with adenoviruses used as gene-therapy vectors, the scientists left in the gene that lets adenoviruses destroy the cells they infect. The plan was for the viruses to infect only the cancer cells and kill them.

Fadlo Khuri, another scientist at the M. D. Anderson Center, began testing the engineered virus, called ONYX-015, in people with head and neck cancers in the late 1990s. Khuri's group announced in August 2000 that in a phase II test the gene therapy, combined with two anticancer drugs, shrank tumors in twenty-five out of thirty patients. They said this was the first phase II test of a cancer gene therapy in which a significant number of tumors vanished and did not return.

Wiping out cancer completely with gene therapy is likely to remain difficult, if not impossible. In theory, the therapy must reach every single cancer cell, because any that escape can start new tumors. No existing technology can assure this. However, gene therapy may make standard cancer treatments such as radiation and chemotherapy more effective, especially in cancers that have not yet spread to distant parts of the body.

Blocking HIV

Researchers are also investigating gene therapy as a way of treating or preventing AIDS. Although new drugs have given people with AIDS a much better chance of long-term survival than they would have had even a few years ago, these are far from ideal treatments. Most patients must take a host of different pills several times a day. The drugs are very expensive, have annoying and sometimes serious side effects, and do not work for all patients. Furthermore, HIV, the retrovirus that causes the disease, often becomes resistant to them.

Some gene therapies for AIDS try to block viral genes named Rev and Tat, which must be active for HIV to reproduce inside cells. One therapy uses what is called antisense DNA. Researchers create short strings of DNA in the laboratory that have a sequence of bases exactly opposite to the sequence in Rev or Tat. They put these pieces of DNA into the kind of immune-system cells that HIV infects. The cells copy each "backward" DNA strand into a single strand of RNA with the same

This model shows the Human Immuno-deficiency Virus (HIV) attacking a cell.

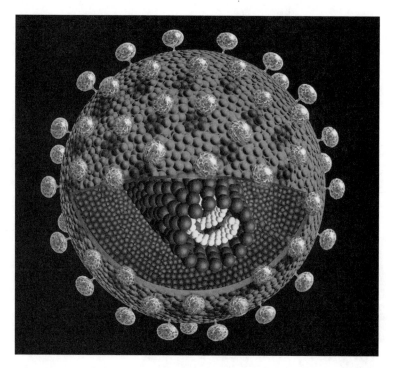

sequence. If HIV enters the cell, this RNA will attach itself to the virus's Rev or Tat gene, just as "sticky ends" bound genes together for the first gene splicers. The gene then cannot function. This treatment has been tested on animals and, to a very limited extent, on the cells of HIV-positive people. As with gene therapy for cancer, this and other gene therapies for AIDS probably would be used along with conventional treatments rather than in place of them.

Heart disease, cancer, and AIDS are just a few of the diseases and medical conditions for which gene therapies are being developed today. Others include diabetes, arthritis, Alzheimer's disease (a disease that breaks down the brains of elderly people), and baldness. All these treatments are still in the early stages of testing and will not be in regular use for at least five or ten years. Many may never be. Still, this wide range of research projects shows clearly that gene therapy has moved far beyond its original goal of replacing defective genes.

CHAPTER 5

A Troubled Industry

Jesse Gelsinger was an energetic eighteen-year-old from Tucson, Arizona, who loved motorcycles and professional wrestling. He let little stand in his way in spite of having been born with a rare disease that kept his liver from breaking down ammonia, a chemical that is poisonous if it builds up in the body. Jesse had a fairly mild form of this illness, called ornithine transcarbamylase deficiency, and drugs and a strict diet kept it under control. Still, when he heard that James Wilson and others at the University of Pennsylvania's Institute for Human Gene Therapy were doing phase I tests of a possible gene therapy for the disease, he was eager to sign up. "He said, 'Hey, this may be good for me, and I'll be helping newborn infants,'"[30] Jesse's father, handyman Paul Gelsinger, remembered later.

On September 13, 1999, researchers injected trillions of adenoviruses carrying the ornithine transcarbamylase gene into the artery leading to Jesse Gelsinger's liver. The ammonia levels in his blood soon began to rise rapidly, showing that his liver was under attack. One by one his organs failed, and on September 17 he died.

Investigators later agreed that the most likely cause of Gelsinger's death was not the gene therapy itself but a massive immune reaction to the virus that carried the genes. Still, if he had not had the treatment, he would not have died. Gelsinger's was the first death that could be blamed directly on gene therapy, and news of it hit the infant medical field like an atomic bomb. "It . . . caught everybody totally off-guard,"[31] French Anderson, then at the University of Southern California, recalled in early 2001. That shock turned out to be just the first of many.

Hype and Hope

Jesse Gelsinger's death was not the first bump in the road for gene therapy. During the 1990s opinions about this new kind of medical treatment had gone through more ups and downs than a roller-coaster ride. At first, after Anderson's success with Ashanthi DeSilva, the roller coaster shot toward the sky. The media, the public, business investors, and even some scientists began to believe that cures for inherited diseases, and perhaps even for such major killers as cancer, were right around the corner. Many gene-therapy researchers founded small biotechnology companies, hoping to gain more funding for their research and also to cash in on the financial bonanzas they thought were sure to result when the new therapies could finally be sold. They became impatient with testing cells and mice and raced to begin trials on human beings.

The results of those first tests, however, were disappointing, and hopes for gene-therapy "miracle cures" began to fade. "There was initially a great burst of enthusiasm that lasted three, four years where a couple of hundred [human] trials got started all over the world," Anderson remembers. "Then we came to realize that nothing was really working at the clinical level [in human patients]."[32]

Critics began saying that gene-therapy researchers were rushing too quickly from the laboratory to the

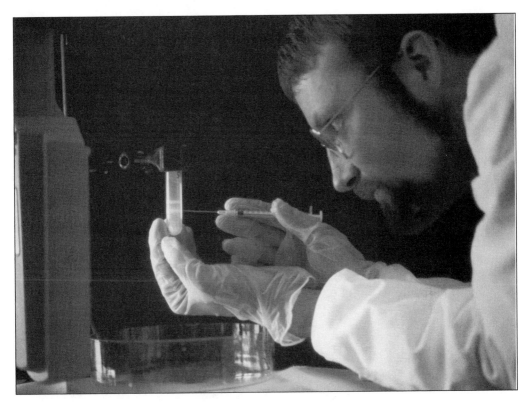

hospital. In December 1995 a panel of scientists appointed by the National Institutes of Health stated that, in its opinion, gene therapy at the moment offered more hype than hope. It told researchers in the field to go back to their labs and do more basic science. Businesspeople began to wonder whether investing in companies that planned to produce and market gene therapies was such a good idea after all.

In the mid-1990s, there was a call to confirm more studies before implementing new-found gene therapies.

Hope slowly returned to the field in the late 1990s, however, as old vectors were improved, new ones were introduced, and some human trials began to produce promising results. At least, people felt, gene therapy was showing itself to be safe. Researchers conducting human trials were supposed to report any serious side effects to both the FDA and the RAC, but few such reports came in.

By 1997, in fact, human tests of gene therapy had become so routine that the FDA and the NIH agreed

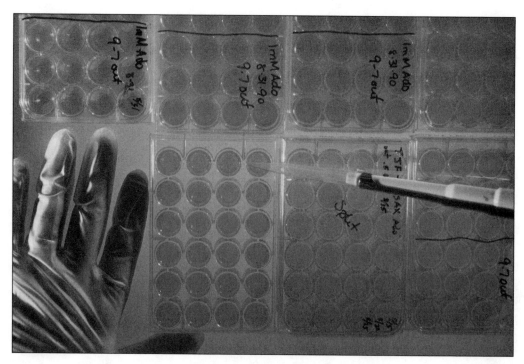

A researcher makes basic preparations of culture dishes.

that only proposals that introduced new technology, such as different vectors, would have to obtain approval from the RAC as well as the FDA before testing began. (All tests still had to be approved by the FDA.) Instead of overseeing test plans, the RAC would hold public hearings on ethical issues related to genetic engineering. According to *Science* magazine, this change reflected feelings that "human gene therapy [had] come of age after a stormy adolescence."[33]

Then Jesse Gelsinger died, and everyone's confidence shattered.

Disturbing Revelations

Not surprisingly, the test that Gelsinger had taken part in was halted at once. The Institute for Human Gene Therapy launched an investigation into his death—and so did the FDA. The agency soon uncovered facts that many people found greatly disturbing. First, FDA investigators claimed in a three-day hearing before the RAC in early December, Gelsinger probably should never have received the gene treatment. Measurements made after he arrived at the hospital had shown a higher level of ammonia in his blood than usual, which meant that his liver was not functioning as well as it normally did. This should have kept him out of the test group. The agency also claimed that the Pennsylvania scientists had not told it about two other patients, treated before Gelsinger, who had suffered liver damage great enough to make the researchers remove them from the trials.

Second, the FDA questioned the completeness of the consent forms that Jesse and his father had been given. These forms were supposed to tell people planning to take part in the tests about any risks that the treatments might have. They were required to list problems that had occurred in earlier tests. The consent forms for this test, however, had included no mention of the two patients who had been removed from the trial or of several monkeys that had died from the treatment. "We gave our consent," Paul Gelsinger said in February 2000, "but in no way was it informed."[34]

The NIH's RAC, meanwhile, put other human gene-therapy tests under its microscope. In early November the committee accused Jeffrey Isner, hailed for his use of gene therapy to grow new blood vessels in people who had had heart attacks, of failing to inform it of the deaths of six people in his experiments. Amy Patterson, head of the NIH Office of Recombinant DNA Activities, emphasized that "even deaths not initially believed to have been caused by the therapy must be reported to the NIH and made public, because often it is not clear until later whether the therapy actually caused the deaths."[35]

The researchers defended themselves as best they could. Wilson, the leader of the group conducting the tests in which Gelsinger had taken part, said at the December 9 RAC meeting that he did not believe that Gelsinger's ammonia levels had been high enough to exclude him from the experiment. Wilson also claimed that he had told the FDA about the two

patients who had had bad reactions to the treatment
before Gelsinger took it. Isner, for his part, said he
had reported the six deaths to the FDA. He believed
that the deaths were caused by the patients' underly-
ing disease, not by the gene treatment. He therefore
had not realized, he claimed, that he had to tell the
RAC about them as well. "There was never any intent
to conceal anything,"[36] he insisted.

The agencies were not impressed. Citing eighteen
violations of procedure in the Gelsinger tests alone,
the FDA put all human tests overseen by the Institute
for Human Gene Therapy on "clinical hold" on
January 21, 2000. This meant that the institute could
not enroll any new patients in tests until the agency
lifted its ban. "Putting everything together, there
appears to be a real problem with how they conducted their day-to-day operations,"[37] said FDA offi-
cial Philip D. Noguchi.

About a month later, the agency put some of
Isner's experiments on hold as well. After further
investigation it sent him a stern warning letter in
May, complaining, for instance, that one patient had
been admitted into his study even though the
researchers knew that the man had a tumor in his
lung. People with cancer were not supposed to be
given Isner's gene treatment because cancers use
growth factors like the one in his therapy to form
their own new blood vessels. Isner's heart therapy
tests remained on hold in mid-2001, but he was testing a similar treatment on people whose leg arteries
have been blocked by disease.

A Wake-Up Call

NIH officials announced that in the future they would
insist on more complete reporting of side effects that
occur during gene-therapy trials. Investigation had
shown, for instance, that in experiments using adenovirus, the type of vector Jesse Gelsinger had been
given, the NIH had been informed immediately of

only 5 percent of the problems that had arisen.

Other groups joined in the rush to question gene therapy. In February the Cystic Fibrosis Foundation and the Muscular Dystrophy Association stopped their support for some projects until further investigations could be made. A Senate subcommittee held hearings during that same month to determine whether the federal government should increase its monitoring of human gene-therapy tests.

Senator Bill Frist of Tennessee said that what the group learned during the hearings "sobered us all."[38] The committee was especially concerned about the fact that many gene-therapy researchers, including Wilson and Isner, were affiliated with biotechnology companies that could profit from the treatments they were testing. This created a potential conflict of interest that might encourage the scientists to exaggerate good results or hide bad ones. Researchers might be especially reluctant to tell the RAC about side effects because reports to the RAC, unlike those to the FDA, are made public.

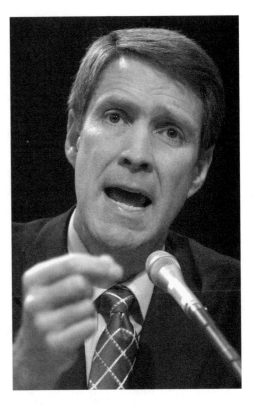

Senator Bill Frist expressed concerns that gene therapists with a stake in biotechnology companies created a conflict of interest, compromising research.

Individuals and groups ranging from drug and biotechnology industry representatives to parents of children with inherited diseases defended gene therapy and urged that human tests continue. Anderson, for example, insisted that "if mistakes were made, they were honest mistakes." But, he admitted, "this is a wake-up call. We have to be more careful."[39]

New Regulations

Many people no longer trusted gene-therapy researchers to heed that wake-up call on their own. In March the administration of President Bill Clinton announced that in the future, all researchers conducting human gene-therapy trials would have to provide the FDA with detailed descriptions of their proposed procedures for monitoring patients' safety. "We see the need to get the concept across that . . . you can't be sloppy when you are dealing with a human," said the FDA's Noguchi. "Everything matters."[40] The NIH, for its part, would hold quarterly public meetings at which gene-therapy researchers could discuss safety, side effects, and other issues.

The University of Pennsylvania, meanwhile, had been conducting its own investigations of the Institute for Human Gene Therapy, which it had sponsored. The university announced in late May that the institute would no longer test gene therapy on humans, although scientists in other departments of the university might do so. Instead, the institute would concentrate on cell and animal research and testing. In December the FDA began proceedings to permanently disqualify the institute's director, James Wilson, from doing human testing in the United States.

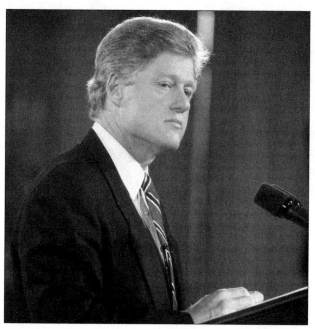

President Bill Clinton required that all gene therapists would have to provide the FDA with detailed descriptions of their proposed procedures.

These were not all of the institute's troubles. A few days after Jesse Gelsinger's death, his father, Paul, had said that the University of Pennsylvania doctors who treated the young man were "good people" and he believed that "their intent was pure."[41] The FDA's findings, however, had made him change his mind. "Jesse was doing the right thing," he told *People Weekly* reporters in February 2000. "Now it looks like he was the only one."[42] In the same month he told the Senate subcommittee, "I am not against gene therapy. I realize it holds so much promise for so many people. But we cannot allow what happened to Jesse to happen again."[43] On September 19, a year and a day after Jesse's death, Paul Gelsinger filed a lawsuit against the people and institutions he held responsible for the tragedy. The suit was settled out of court in November.

In January 2001 the FDA announced that it planned to make public more information about ongoing gene-therapy trials than it had before. This includes records of safety testing, the consent forms used in the trials, and any problems that arise. Most gene-therapy researchers seem to accept this new openness. A report from the FDA in April stated that further investigation of gene-therapy tests had uncovered relatively few violations—fewer, in fact, than in trials of more standard new drugs or treatments. Joseph Salewski, head of an FDA unit that conducts inspections of human therapy trials, said that researchers were "doing a fairly decent job . . . following protocol [proper procedure] and taking care of patients' rights."[44] The report also said that the scientists seemed to be boosting their efforts to comply with the new government guidelines.

Some commentators think that procedures for human testing could be improved still further, however. Many feel, for instance, that gene therapy should be tested only on people who are terminally or at least severely ill—people who have little or nothing to lose if the treatments fail or cause harm. They have also urged that researchers provide more information to patients before they consent to take part in tests, including any connections the scientists have with for-profit companies. Indeed, the American Society of Gene Therapy, the field's largest professional organization, says that scientists conducting human trials should not even have such ties. In May 2000 the group announced a new policy that "all investigators and team members directly responsible for patient selection, the informed consent process and/or clinical management in a trial must not have equity, stock options or comparable arrangements in companies sponsoring the trial."[45]

The Best and Worst of Times

Even during gene therapy's darkest days, the news was not all bad. News about the French babies whose rare immune-system disorder had been substantially improved, for instance, appeared in April 2000. Commenting in *Science* magazine about both that advance and the Gelsinger case, Anderson borrowed the opening phrase from Charles Dickens's novel about the French Revolution, *A Tale of Two Cities*, to call this period in the history of gene therapy "the best of times, the worst of times." Even the FDA's Noguchi admitted in September that "there is good progress being made. FDA thinks that gene therapy will work."[46]

Indeed, there has been plenty of evidence that the shock waves produced by Jesse Gelsinger's death did not shut down gene-therapy research. *Fortune* magazine reported in May 2000 that in the months since Gelsinger had died, the NIH had received more than fifty proposals for new gene-therapy tests—40 percent more than in the same period during the previous year. Even as some researchers' tests were temporarily or permanently halted, other groups continued their investigations of similar treatments. Some scientists even feel that, in the long run, the shake-up that resulted from Gelsinger's death helped the gene-therapy industry. Paul Fischer, president of GenVec of Gaithersburg, Maryland—one of several biotechnology companies working on gene therapy for heart disease—said in early 2001, "As tragic as that event [Gelsinger's death] was, I think it helped people understand how to move forward in the future safely and carefully. It made people double-check the safety issue."[47]

Researchers today are exploring new techniques to make gene therapy both safer and more effective. For instance, Michael Blaese, who left the NIH in 1998 to become chief scientific officer of a Pennsylvania biotechnology company called Kimeragen, is investigating a way to repair damaged genes rather than replacing them. Named chimeraplasty after the "patchwork monster" of Greek legend, this technique inserts short pieces of an artificial combination of RNA and DNA that attach to particular genetic flaws. The added pieces give the cell instructions for correcting the mistakes. "All it does is change [the defective gene's] spelling,"[48] Blaese says.

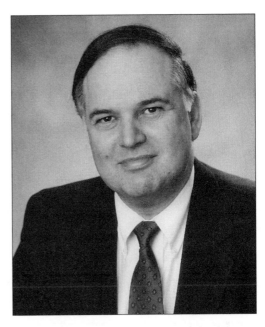

Michael Blaese, chief scientific officer of Kimeragen, is investigating a way to repair damaged genes rather than replacing them.

Judging Gene Therapy

Scientists and the public remain divided in their opinions of gene therapy. Critics point not only to Jesse Gelsinger's death and the disturbing discoveries that followed it, but to the fact that, more than ten years after altered cells began flowing into little Ashi DeSilva's arm, gene therapy has not yet provided an unquestioned cure or even a consistently dependable treatment for any disease or medical condition. "I have been very disappointed"[49] with gene therapy's progress, said Abbey S. Meyers, president of the National Organization for Rare Disorders, Inc., in 2000.

Supporters of this new field, on the other hand, remind critics that most tests of gene therapy so far have been phase I tests. Such tests are designed to examine primarily the safety of treatments, not their effectiveness. They point to the fact that in some four hundred trials involving about six thousand patients worldwide, Gelsinger's is the only death definitely shown to have been caused by the therapy or a reaction to it—not a bad safety record for a wholly new treatment. They also note that most new drugs or other treatments, let alone those as revolutionary as gene therapy, take at least ten years to develop. Gene therapy is in its infancy, its believers say, and it should be given a chance to grow up before it is judged.

The one thing that both critics and supporters agree on is that gene therapy will not become a regular treatment for many diseases—perhaps for any—for at least five years, quite possibly ten or twenty. Many more discoveries must be made and many more tests must be undergone before results will be clear. Patients looking for cures and biotechnology companies looking for profits will both have to wait. As

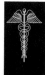

New Views of the Gene

In basic research that is sure to affect gene therapy, scientists are arriving at new understandings of what a gene is and how it works. Nathaniel C. Comfort descibes this and other research on genes in "Are Genes Real?"—an article published in Natural History *in June 2001.*

In 1977 two research groups, one led by Richard Roberts at Cold Spring Harbor Laboratory and the other led by Phillip Sharp at MIT, found that the many DNA segments that constitute a single gene are sometimes quite distantly separated on the chromosome. In such genes the segments are then spliced together to compose the RNA message. Furthermore, the same segments can be combined in different ways, which means that one gene is capable of specifying a whole family of products: one gene, sometimes several enzymes.

And the story gets even more complicated. Biologists have found examples of genes within genes and even overlapping genes. In some cases, the same DNA sequence specifies one protein when read in the "forward" direction and another when read "in reverse." Muddling things further, the instructions encoded in the DNA do not always reach the ribosome [the part of the cell in which proteins are made] as a literal translation. In a phenomenon known as RNA editing, an enzymatic highwayman [bandit] intercepts the RNA message en route and alters it, so the resulting protein is not identical to that specified by the DNA. . . .

DNA is not made of discrete [separate] units with fixed boundaries; it comprises [is made up of] great lengths of sequence that are altered, shuffled, and reused.

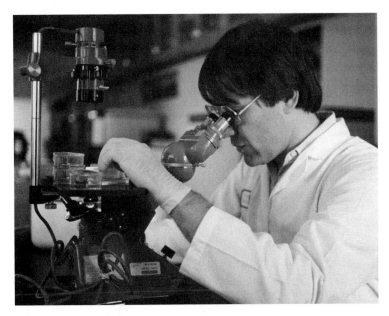

Many more tests must be confirmed before genetic therapy will become regular treatments.

Eduardo Aguilar of the Baylor College of Medicine in Houston, Texas, says:

> The way I like to think about it is that we've finished Chapter One of a very long book. We've had the introduction, the expectations out of line with reality, and a tremendous amount of hype. Now we're seeing a closure to Chapter One and we're beginning Chapter Two, this time with more realistic expectations.[50]

Meanwhile, other commentators are asking even harder questions than those raised by Jesse Gelsinger's death. Important as safety is, it is far from the only ethical issue that gene therapy raises. Some ethicists are starting to think about what might happen in twenty or thirty years if, as gene therapy's boosters predict, alteration of human genes becomes a fairly routine medical treatment. In that case, gene therapy—and alteration of genes that goes beyond therapy—could change the definitions of health, disease, and even perhaps humanity itself.

CHAPTER 6

The Ethics of Gene Therapy

University of Pennsylvania researcher H. Lee Sweeney has been testing a new gene treatment in mice. He injects the animals' muscles with viruses carrying the gene for a substance called insulinlike growth factor-1 (IGF-1). This protein makes the muscles grow larger than average and heal more quickly after injury. It even prevents the weakness that normally develops in the muscles of mice—and humans—as a result of age. An elderly mouse that had received the treatment in its youth had a muscle mass 60 percent greater than that of a normal mouse of the same age. "We showed that with a onetime injection of this gene we can get bigger muscles in young animals and that, as they get older, the muscles never change,"[51] Sweeney told *Sports Illustrated* reporters in 2001.

As of mid-2001 Sweeney had no immediate plans to test his treatment on humans. Nonetheless, he was already hearing from volunteers who were eager to let him give it to them. They were not the muscular dystrophy patients or elderly people for whom he had designed the therapy. Instead, they were athletes who hoped that the treatment would give them an extra edge in sports contests. Sweeney said that as far as these athletes were concerned, "the main question was how could they get it. I told them I had no safety data on humans whatsoever, but . . . they were fine with that. Safety data didn't mean anything to them. They basically said they were willing to do it right now."[52]

Sweeney is not accepting any of these volunteers. The fact that they sought him out, however, highlights one of the main ethical challenges that researchers and, eventually, ordinary doctors will face if gene therapy ever becomes routine: deciding who should receive it and why. Few people would doubt the morality of altering human genes to treat or prevent life-threatening or seriously disabling illness. Critics fear, however, that even this use might

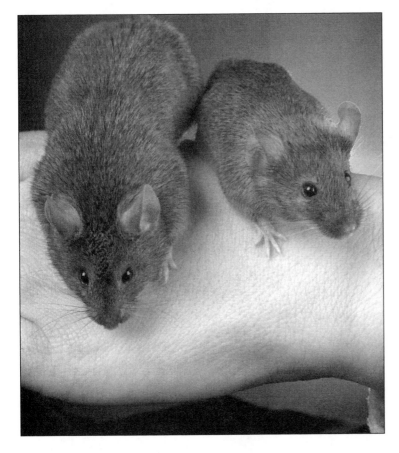

Some athletes would like to have the gene treatment that made the muscles of the mouse on the left larger and stronger.°

start society down a "slippery slope" toward much more questionable genetic changes.

The Ethics of Immortality

Athletes altering their genes to gain an advantage in competition are not the only people who might use gene therapy in ethically doubtful ways. What if, as many gene-therapy researchers predict, gene treatments make it possible for people to live in good health for 150 years or more? Would it be ethical for people to take advantage of such "immortality"?

Some observers see gene therapy to halt or reverse aging as merely another step in the advancement of medicine that has already made life spans almost twice what they were in earlier centuries. To be sure, such therapy, like most new treatments, would probably be very expensive at first. It therefore would be available only to the wealthy. That would not necessarily make it unethical, says British bioethicist John Harris. "We do not refuse kidney transplants to some patients because we cannot provide them for all, nor do we regard ourselves as wicked because we [in

Gene therapy, which may allow people to live beyond natural life expectancy, raises many ethical issues.

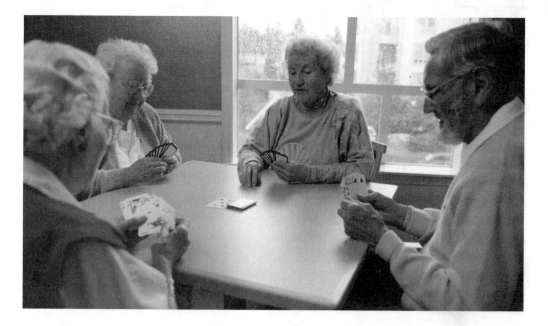

wealthy countries] perform many such transplants, while low-income countries perform few or none at all,"[53] Harris points out.

On the other hand, some ethicists say, people should think about the social effects that individual medical decisions can have. The world is already overcrowded. If large numbers of people begin living for a very long time, writes eminent biologist Edward O. Wilson, society could change in some startling ways:

> The first thing people will have to do is virtually stop having children. . . . We may reach a point when it becomes a high privilege to be able to have a child or to provide the DNA for a new child. . . . The species is likely to end up with people who have the physical capabilities of teenagers but who are culturally, educationally, and emotionally aged. It's likely to be a very conservative culture, one in which those who have survived and enjoyed longevity [life-span] extension . . . won't be revolutionaries. They won't be bold entrepreneurs [creators of new businesses] or explorers who risk their lives. . . . [Extended life is] too precious a gift.[54]

Treating Unborn Children

Even greater ethical questions will arise if gene therapy is applied to children, especially those not yet born. French Anderson, for one, is already planning to use gene therapy on babies in the womb. Tests of cells in the fluid that surrounds the unborn child, or fetus, can identify a number of genetic defects, including ADA deficiency, the condition Ashanthi DeSilva has. Anderson told the RAC in 1998 that if animal tests showed that the procedure appeared to be safe and effective, he would ask for permission to do gene therapy on fetuses shown to have ADA deficiency or another genetic blood disease.

Treating fetuses has advantages over giving therapy after birth, Anderson claims. Such treatment could prevent the often serious and irreversible harm that the defect would cause by the time of birth or shortly thereafter. In the case of ADA deficiency, for instance, it could prevent the damage that infections do to the bodies of immune-weakened children. Giving gene therapy to fetuses might also be safer and more effective than giving it to children or adults because a fetus's immune system is not yet fully developed. It therefore would be unlikely to have the kind of overreaction to gene-carrying viruses that killed Jesse Gelsinger.

If such a treatment could be shown to be safe, most people probably would see nothing wrong with "fixing" a fetus's genes to prevent a life-threatening or disabling illness, especially if such treatment would provide an alternative to aborting the fetus. Indeed, says James Watson, codiscoverer of DNA's structure and one of genetic engineering's most energetic boosters, in a world of safe and effective gene therapy for fetuses, society might decide that it is "true moral cowardice to allow children to be born with known genetic defects."[55] But what exactly will be considered to be a defect? As Sheldon Krimsky, a professor of science policy at Boston's Tufts University, says, "We know where to start [with gene therapy]—but do we know where to stop?"[56]

Performing genetic treatment on unborn fetuses could rouse even greater ethical debates.

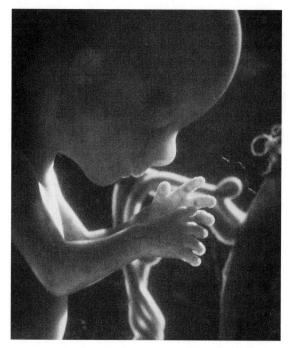

Going Beyond Health

Many people question how much control parents should have over their children's genes. Should they be allowed to choose (or alter) a child's sex, eye or hair color, or skin color? Should they be permitted to remove genes that might make a child, say, unusually short or fat? Should they be able to add genes that give a child a better memory or stronger muscles?

The question of whether parents should have the right to ask for a treatment that adds a quality to healthy children rather than remedying problems suffered by sick ones has already surfaced, although the treatment in question did not alter genes. This ethical issue arose in the 1980s, when use of genetically engineered bacteria made human growth hormone available in relatively large amounts for the first time.

Before that time, when growth hormone could be obtained only in tiny amounts, it was used mainly to treat children who had been born without the power to make their own supply. These children were extremely short and also suffered other physical problems. After the hormone became more widely available, however, the parents of some healthy children began demanding it as well. Their children had normal amounts of growth hormone, but they were shorter than average. The parents believed that short people receive less respect and are less likely to be successful in life than tall people, and they wanted to help the children avoid this situation. Some ethicists fear that future parents might similarly request gene therapy for traits that cause no real health problem but simply meet with society's disapproval.

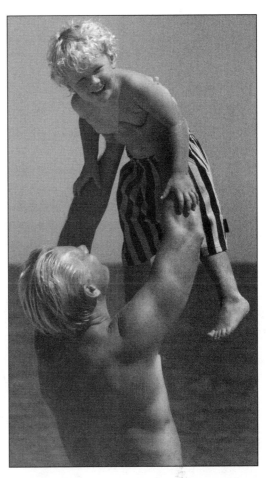

Manipulating a healthy child's genes for more desirable traits poses an ethical dilemma.

Several ethical objections have been made to allowing genetic enhancement of children—treatments that add genes to improve normal traits such as memory or remove genes associated with characteristics that do not cause serious health problems, such as shortness or nearsightedness. Some critics say that being able to specify genes for "designer babies" would make parents think of children more as products to be ordered out of a catalog than as independent beings. It could "come very close to turning human procreation [reproduction] into manufacture,"[57] says University of Chicago bioethicist Leon Kass. It also forces competition for money and prestige to begin even earlier in life than it does today, when some parents begin preparing a child to go to a particular college or follow a particular career while the child is still in nursery school. Philip Kitcher, a bioethics professor at Columbia University in New York, calls it "putting the rat race into the womb."[58]

Some commentators say that letting parents choose genes to enhance their children is unethical because the unborn children have no say in those choices. If parents give children names that the children hate, they can change them after they grow up. They could not easily do that with changes in their genes. UCLA geneticist John Campbell suggests an interesting way around this particular problem, however. Just as is proposed for certain gene therapies now, he says, optional genes could be constructed so that they would turn on only when a person takes a certain drug. When engineered children reach adulthood, they could be told about the advantages and disadvantages of the genes their parents chose. They would then decide whether to take the drug that activated the genes.

There is also the danger that, rather than working to eliminate society's prejudices against people with certain characteristics, parents would simply try to help their children

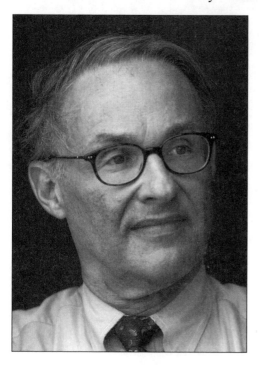

Dr. Leon Kass is calling for guidelines and regulations in genetic treatment.

avoid those prejudices by changing genes that determine, say, skin color. This could reduce diversity and respect for other people's differences. Relatedly, the fact that, at least at first, only the wealthy would be able to afford gene enhancement might widen the present social gap between rich and poor. Because the ethics of gene enhancement are so doubtful, Anderson believes that "we should not use human genetic engineering for any other purpose than the treatment of serious disease, no matter how tempting it might be."[59]

Not everyone sees gene enhancement as unethical, though. Supporters of this extension of gene therapy say that most parents already try to gain all the advantages for their children that they can. The rich usually can obtain more, such as better clothes or schooling. There is no reason, these supporters say, why improving the genes of unborn children should be any less ethical than, say, sending children to an expensive private school. "If you're not taking any [health] risks, then it's hard to criticize the goal of trying to biologically make your child better,"[60] says Arthur Caplan, a bioethicist at the University of Pennsylvania. According to a 1998 March of Dimes survey, more than 40 percent of those surveyed in the United States and Britain saw nothing wrong with gene enhancement.

Changing Future Generations

The ethical questions will become even greater if scientists become able and willing to alter the genes that are passed on to offspring—the so-called germline genes. They can do this now in animals, and fetal treatments such as the one Anderson is proposing carry a small risk of changing human germline genes accidentally. All gene therapies tried so far produce changes only in the genomes of somatic, or body, cells: cells other than sex cells. Such treatments change genes in blood cells or muscle cells, for example. Because the added genes do not enter the sex cells, they are not passed on to a person's off-spring. Changes in germline genes, however, would be inherited by the person's children—and grandchildren, great-grandchildren, and so on through the generations. A mistake in gene therapy affecting somatic cells could ruin one life, but a mistake in germline gene therapy could ruin many. Because of this, altering germline genes is much more controversial than altering the genes of somatic cells.

It might seem hard to question the ethics of removing a defective gene known to cause a serious or

Selecting Embryos

Some scientists and ethicists say that germline genes do not need to be altered, even to prevent inherited diseases, because a technique already exists to let parents avoid giving birth to a child with such a disease. It is called embryo selection.

In this technique, parents who carry a disease-causing gene provide eggs and sperm, which are combined at a fertility clinic to make fertilized eggs. Several of these eggs are allowed to divide in the clinic's laboratory until they produce clusters of eight or six-teen cells each. These clusters are very early forms of embryos, living things that have just started to develop. (Unborn humans are considered to be embryos for the first two months of their development. After that they are called fetuses.) Technicians can remove a single cell from each cluster without harming the embryo. They analyze the DNA in the cells to find out which embryos have two copies of the defective gene and therefore would inherit the disease. Only healthy embryos will be placed in the mother's uterus and allowed to develop further. The others are discarded.

To be sure, some people say that destroying embryos is the same as abortion, which they feel is morally wrong. However, supporters of embryo selection as an alternative to germline gene therapy say that embryos would probably be destroyed in gene therapy too, because the therapy most likely would fail in some of the fertilized eggs in which it was tried.

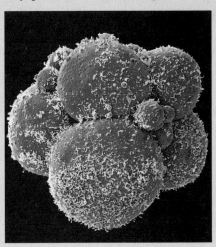

An eight-cell embryo.

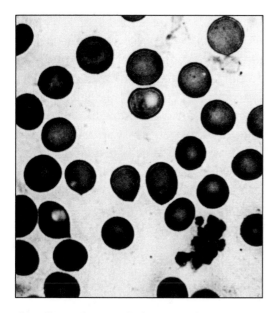 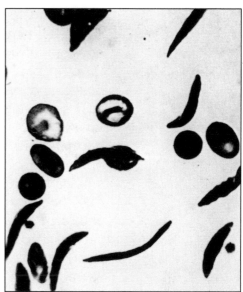

These slides show normal red blood cells (left) and cells deformed by sickle-cell anemia (right).

deadly inherited disease from an entire family line. Doing so would certainly seem more efficient, less expensive, and safer than having to treat each individual born (or conceived) with the disease. Some scientists and ethicists do feel that this kind of germline therapy is ethical. Others, however, point to the fact that scientists know very little about what individual genes do. They know even less about the complex ways in which genes interact with one another and with people's environment. This means that in removing a gene with a known harmful effect, they might also permanently destroy a beneficial effect that had not yet been recognized.

Researchers already know about one gene that can have both harmful and helpful effects. It is the gene that causes sickle-cell anemia, a serious blood disease that can affect people of African descent. Like most genes that cause inherited diseases, the sickle-cell gene is recessive. People who inherit copies of it from both parents have the disease and, until recently, usually did not live long enough to have children. Scientists wondered, therefore, why this gene had not died out of the population long ago.

In fact, there seems to be a good reason why the sickle-cell gene has persisted. People who inherit just one copy of this gene, along with a normal copy from the other parent, are perfectly healthy. Indeed, scientists have found that these people—called sickle-cell carriers, or possessors of sickle-cell trait—are more likely to survive in their homeland than people who inherit two normal copies of the gene. This is because a single copy of the gene somehow helps blood cells resist the microscopic parasites that cause malaria, a serious blood disease that produces repeated attacks of fever, weakness, and often death. Malaria, which is spread by the bite of certain mosquitoes, is very common in Africa. Removing the sickle-cell gene from the germline would spare future generations the pain of sickle-cell anemia, but it would also remove this useful resistance.

Many gene researchers believe that other genes that cause fairly common inherited diseases may have similar "good sides." It would be foolish, they say, to remove these or any other genes permanently without knowing more about what they do. Because genes interact with one another in complex ways, adding or subtracting germline genes could have dangerous effects that would reveal themselves only several generations after the changes were made.

A New Eugenics?

The ethical questions raised by the creation of "designer babies"—gene enhancement—become even greater when the design is being applied not just to an individual child, but to all of his or her future descendants. Many critics of germline gene alteration fear that it would lead to a new form of a now-discarded doctrine called eugenics. The term, which means "well born," was coined in the late nineteenth century by Francis Galton, a cousin of Charles Darwin. Galton had noticed that not only physical characteristics but some psychological ones, such as intelligence, tended to run in families. He stated that the quality of the human race could be improved if people who possessed desirable characteristics were encouraged to have children and those with undesirable characteristics were discouraged from doing so.

There are a number of problems with Galton's idea. First, complex characteristics such as intelligence are sure to be affected by many different genes. These genes, furthermore, interact in complicated ways with environmental factors such as schooling. Thus, although two intelligent parents would be more likely to have intelligent children than two parents of lesser intelligence, no particular results could be guaranteed.

The second problem is that choices of "desirable" characteristics—or even definitions of traits like intelligence—are shaped far more by social and cultural beliefs than by science. Galton focused on characteristics that were valued by his social group, upper-class white Englishmen. The characteristics he called undesirable were often associated with people of other classes, cultures, or ethnic groups.

Belief in eugenics led to serious abuses of human rights. In the early twentieth century, state or national governments in Canada, the United States, and several other countries forcibly sterilized (made unable to reproduce) people who were considered undesirable, such as those with a severe mental illness or developmental disability. The leaders of Nazi Germany carried negative eugenics (keeping people with "bad" traits from reproducing) to its ultimate extreme in the late 1930s. They used eugenic doctrine as a reason for not merely sterilizing but killing members of groups they considered undesirable, especially Jews.

If a particular social group controlled germline gene alteration, critics say, they might be able to inflict their tastes

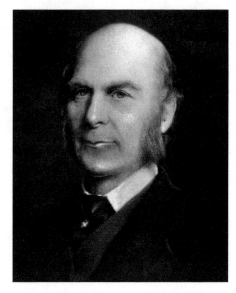

Francis Galton first introduced the idea of eugenics.

and prejudices on others to a far greater degree than even the Nazis could. At worst, they might carry out true genocide, the complete destruction of a race or ethnic group. Even if that did not happen, allowing the fashions and beliefs of a particular era to dictate the nature of humanity for many generations to come could produce unpredictable and possibly disastrous effects. Leon Kass writes:

During the 1930s, Hitler and the Nazi regime sterilized and killed millions in an extreme promotion of eugenics.

> It will not do to assert that we can extrapolate [extend our reasoning] from what we like about ourselves. Because memory is good, can we say how much more memory would be better? If sexual desire is good, how much more would be better? Life is good; but how much extension of life would be good for us? Only sim-

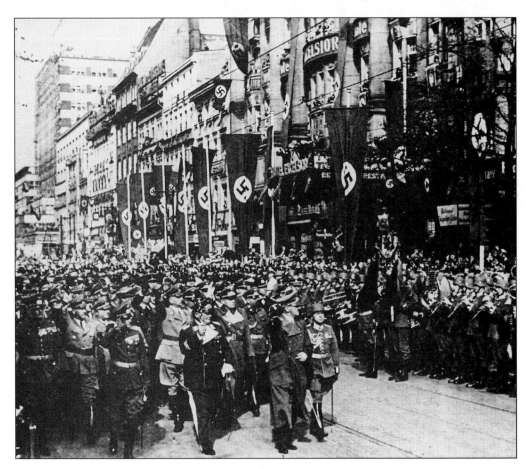

plistic thinkers believe they can easily answer such questions.[61]

Some scientists, such as Princeton University microbiologist Lee Silver, have predicted that wealthy parents' use of germline gene enhancement will eventually divide humanity into two different species. Silver terms them the "gen-rich" and the "naturals." He does not think that such a change would necessarily be bad, but his vision of a genetically divided society frightens many.

Deciding About Gene Therapy

Many gene-therapy scientists feel that no changes should be made in human germline genes, at least until much more is understood about how genes work—and perhaps ever. Some governments, such as the European Union, have made germline gene alteration illegal. These individuals and groups, along with many others, believe that germline gene alteration presents great potential threats, not only to the rights of individuals but to large groups and even, perhaps, humanity as a whole.

Others are less sure. Even religious groups, which have often questioned the ethics of genetic engineering, do not necessarily rule out germline gene alteration. "There is no prohibition in the Roman Catholic Church against inherited genetic modification,"[62] says Albert S. Moraczeski, president emeritus of the National Catholic Bioethics Center. Similarly, Laurie Zoloth, chair of the Jewish studies program in the College of Humanities at San Francisco State University, says that "religious traditions are alert to the possibility that any type of medicine . . . can be used for good or evil," but this is no reason "to turn away from a healing intervention"[63] in the form of changing germline genes. Some of gene therapy's most enthusiastic supporters, such as James Watson, even see nothing wrong with humans trying to direct their own evolution.

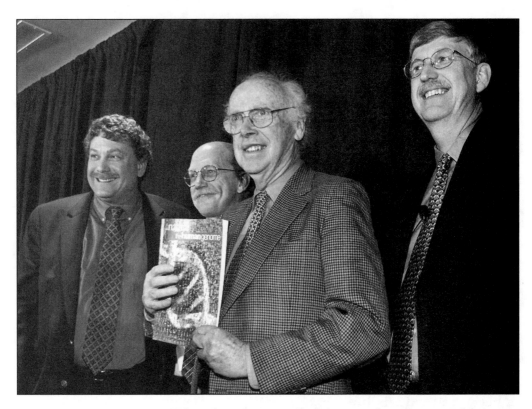

One of gene therapy's most enthusiastic supporters, Dr. James Watson (holding magazine) poses after announcing the sequencing of the human genome.

Ethical questions about gene therapy—and human gene alteration that goes beyond therapy—are sure to produce passionate discussion during the coming decades, not only among scientists but among members of the public. Most gene-therapy researchers and bioethicists think that is exactly what should happen. "Unless we mobilize the courage to look foursquare at the full human meaning of our new enterprise in biogenetic technology and engineering," says Kass, "we are doomed to become its creatures if not its slaves."[64]

NOTES

Introduction: Gene Therapy: A New Medical Frontier

1. Jeff Lyon and Peter Gorner, *Altered Fates: Gene Therapy and the Retooling of Human Life*. New York: W. W. Norton, 1996, p. 28.
2. Quoted in Lyon and Gorner, *Altered Fates*, p. 35.

Chapter 1: Deadly Legacies

3. Quoted in Colin Tudge, *The Engineer in the Garden: Genes and Genetics: From the Idea of Heredity to the Creation of Life*. London: Jonathan Cape, 1993, p. 4.
4. Quoted in Tudge, *The Engineer in the Garden*, p. 65.
5. Quoted in Walter Bodmer and Robin McKie, *The Book of Man*. New York: Scribner's, 1994, p. 43.

Chapter 2: The Birth of Gene Therapy

6. Quoted in Lyon and Gorner, *Altered Fates*, p. 21.
7. Quoted in Lyon and Gorner, *Altered Fates*, p. 168.
8. Quoted in Lyon and Gorner, *Altered Fates*, p. 168.
9. Quoted in Lyon and Gorner, *Altered Fates*, p. 205.
10. Quoted in Lyon and Gorner, *Altered Fates*, p. 210.
11. Quoted in Joseph Levine and David Suzuki, *The Secret of Life*. Boston: WGBH Educational Foundation, 1993, p. 207.

Chapter 3: Repairing Damaged Genes

12. W. French Anderson, "Gene Therapy," *Scientific American*, September 1995, p. 124.

13. Quoted in *Business Week*, "Gene Therapy: One Family's Story," July 12, 1999, p. 94.
14. Quoted in *Business Week*, "Gene Therapy," p. 94.
15. Quoted in Leon Jaroff, "Fixing the Genes," *Time*, January 11, 1999, p. 68.
16. Quoted in Tom Abate, "Possible Leap Forward for Hemophiliacs," *San Francisco Chronicle*, April 12, 1999, p. B1.
17. Quoted in Muscular Dystrophy Association, "New Hope for Gene Therapy of DMD, BMD Using AAV Vectors," *MDA/Quest*, August 2000, www.mdausa.org/publications/Quest/q74resup.html#newhope.
18. *Business Week*, "Score One for Gene Therapy," May 8, 2000, p. 58.
19. Quoted in Jaroff, "Fixing the Genes," pp. 68 ff.

Chapter 4: Treating Common Killers

20. Quoted in Patrick Perry, "The Coronary Gene Therapy Program," *Saturday Evening Post*, March 2000, p. 39.
21. Quoted in Jaroff, "Fixing the Genes," pp. 68 ff.
22. Quoted in Jaroff, "Fixing the Genes," pp. 68 ff.
23. Quoted in *Saturday Evening Post*, "The Stokes Family Saga," May 2000, pp. 42 ff.
24. Quoted in Cory SerVaas and Patrick Perry, "Coronary Gene Therapy: Restoring Hope and Lives," *Saturday Evening Post*, May 2000, p. 38.
25. Quoted in Rick Weiss, "Gene Therapy Benefits Cited; Study Suggests Diseased Heart Cells Renewed; Doubts Remain," *Washington Post*, August 29, 2000, p. A2.
26. Quoted in Jeff Goldberg, "A Head Full of Hope," *Discover*, April 1998, p. 73.
27. Quoted in Goldberg, "A Head Full of Hope," p. 73.
28. Quoted in Goldberg, "A Head Full of Hope," pp. 75–76.

29. Quoted in Helen Thorpe, "Jack Roth: He's Helping Solve One of Medicine's Biggest Mysteries: Cancer. It's All in the Genes," *Texas Monthly*, September 1998, p. 132.

Chapter 5: A Troubled Industry

30. Quoted in Angie Cannon, "Humility at the Frontier," *U.S. News & World Report*, December 20, 1999, p. 60.
31. Quoted in Terence Chea, "Gene Therapy's Hot Seat: Ignoring Skeptics, GenVec Forges Ahead with Drug Development," *Washington Post*, February 20, 2001, p. E1.
32. Quoted in Larry Thompson, "Human Gene Therapy: Harsh Lessons, High Hopes," *FDA Consumer*, September 2000, p. 19.
33. Eliot Marshall, "One Less Hoop for Gene Therapy," *Science*, July 29, 1994, p. 599.
34. Quoted in J. Madeleine Nash, "The Bad and the Good: Fresh Doubts Are Cast on a Troubled Gene-Therapy Experiment Even as the French Hint at New Advances," *Time*, February 14, 2000, p. 67.
35. Quoted in Deborah Nelson and Rick Weiss, "Gene-Experiment Deaths Confirmed by Researchers," *Washington Post*. Reprinted in *San Francisco Chronicle*, November 3, 1999, p. A14.
36. Quoted in Tom Abate, "Death Reports Spark No Cries for Demise of Gene Therapy Studies," *San Francisco Chronicle*, November 8, 1999, p. B1.
37. Quoted in *Washington Post*, "Probe of Death Prompts Halt to Penn's Gene Tests." Reprinted in *San Francisco Chronicle*, January 22, 2000.
38. Quoted in Richard Jerome, Jerry Kammer, and Matt Birkbeck, "Death by Research: A Teenager's Death in a Clinical Trial Raises Questions About Gene Therapy's Future," *People Weekly*, February 21, 2000, pp. 123 ff.

39. Quoted in Cannon, "Humility at the Frontier," p. 60.
40. Quoted in Thompson, "Human Gene Therapy," pp. 19 ff.
41. Quoted in Leslie Roberts, "A Promising Experiment Ends in Tragedy," *U.S. News & World Report*, October 11, 1999, p. 43.
42. Quoted in Jerome et al., "Death by Research," pp. 123 ff.
43. Quoted in Nash, "The Bad and the Good," p. 67.
44. Quoted in *San Francisco Chronicle*, "Gene Trials Show Few Violations, FDA Audit Says," April 9, 2001.
45. American Society of Gene Therapy, "Position/Policy Statement on Financial Conflict of Interest in Clinical Research." www.asgt.org/policy.
46. Quoted in Thompson, "Human Gene Therapy," pp. 19 ff.
47. Quoted in Chea, "Gene Therapy's Hot Seat," p. E1.
48. Quoted in Trisha Gura, "Repairing the Genome's Spelling Mistakes," *Science*, July 16, 1999, p. 316.
49. Quoted in Thompson, "Human Gene Therapy," p. 19.
50. Quoted in Nash, "The Bad and the Good," p. 67.

Chapter 6: The Ethics of Gene Therapy

51. Quoted in E. M. Swift and Don Yeager, "Unnatural Selection," *Sports Illustrated*, May 14, 2001, p. 86.
52. Quoted in Swift and Yeager, "Unnatural Selection," pp. 86 ff.
53. John Harris, "Intimations of Immortality," *Science*, April 7, 2000, p. 59.
54. Edward O. Wilson, "A World of Immortal Men," *Esquire*, May 1999, p. 84.
55. Quoted in Joannie Fischer, "Passing on Perfection," *U.S. News & World Report*, October 2, 2000, p. 54.
56. Quoted in Sharon Begley, "Designer Babies," *Newsweek*, November 9, 1998, p. 61.
57. Leon R. Kass, "The Moral Meaning of Genetic Technology," *Commentary*, September 1999, pp. 32 ff.

58. Quoted in Amy Otchet, "The Dangers of Laissez Faire Eugenics," *UNESCO Courier*, September 1999, p. 27.

59. French Anderson, "A Cure That May Cost Us Ourselves," *Newsweek*, January 1, 2000, p. 74.

60. Quoted in Otchet, "The Dangers of Laissez Faire Eugenics," p. 27.

61. Kass, "The Moral Meaning of Genetic Technology," pp. 32 ff.

62. Quoted in *Christian Century*, "Study Cites Dangers in Modifying Genes," October 25, 2000, p. 1,065.

63. Quoted in *Christian Century*, "Study Cites Dangers in Modifying Genes," p. 1,065.

64. Kass, "The Moral Meaning of Genetic Technology," pp. 32 ff.

FOR FURTHER READING

Books

William R. Clark, *The New Healers: The Promise and Problems of Molecular Medicine in the Twenty-First Century.* New York: Oxford University Press, 1997. Describes the history, present status, and predicted future of gene therapy.

Jeff Lyon and Peter Gorner, *Altered Fates: Gene Therapy and the Retooling of Human Life.* New York: W. W. Norton, 1996. Describes the first tests of gene therapy on human beings and the events that led up to them.

Jeremy Rifkin, *The Biotech Century: Harnessing the Gene and Remaking the World.* New York: Putnam, 1998. Describes possible dangers of genetic engineering, including alteration of human genes.

Lee M. Silver, *Remaking Eden: How Genetic Engineering and Cloning Will Transform the American Family.* New York: Avon, 1998. Presents a positive view of a future shaped by alteration of human genes.

James D. Torr, ed., *Opposing Viewpoints: Genetic Engineering.* San Diego: Greenhaven Press, 2001. Anthology of articles includes sections on the effects of genetic engineering on society, the regulation of genetic engineering, and the ethics of altering human genes.

Colin Tudge, *The Engineer in the Garden: Genes and Genetics: From the Idea of Heredity to the Creation of Life.* London: Jonathan Cape, 1993. History of genetics and genetic engineering.

Lisa Yount, *Milestones in Discovery and Invention: Genetics and Genetic Engineering.* New York: Facts On File, 1997. Biographies of scientists who shaped these fields, including French Anderson, for young adults.

————, ed. *At Issue: The Ethics of Genetic Engineering.* San Diego: Greenhaven Press, 2001. Short anthology focuses on ethics of altering human genes.

Periodicals

Paul R. Billings, Ruth Hubbard, and Stuart A. Newman, "Human Germline Gene Modification: A Dissent," *Lancet*, May 29, 1999.

Kathryn S. Brown, "Mending Broken Genes," *Popular Science*, October 1999.

Business Week, "Gene Therapy: One Family's Story," July 12, 1999.

Nathaniel C. Comfort, "Are Genes Real?" *Natural History*, June 2001.

Sally Deneen, "Designer People," *E*, January 2001.

Bernard Gert, "Genetic Engineering: Is It Morally Acceptable?" *USA Today Magazine*, January 1999.

Jeff Goldberg, "A Head Full of Hope," *Discover*, April 1998.

Leon Jaroff, "Fixing the Genes," *Time*, January 11, 1999.

Richard Jerome, Jerry Kammer, and Matt Birkbeck, "Death by Research: A Teenager's Death in a Clinical Trial Raises Questions About Gene Therapy's Future," *People Weekly*, February 21, 2000.

Ronald L. Nagel, "Molecule, Heal Thyself," *Natural History*, September 2000.

J. Madeleine Nash, "The Bad and the Good: Fresh Doubts Are Cast on a Troubled Gene-Therapy Treatment Even as the French Hint at New Advances," *Time*, February 14, 2000.

Newsweek, "A Revolution in Medicine: The Search for Cures," April 10, 2000.

Patrick Perry, "The Coronary Gene Therapy Program," *Saturday Evening Post*, March 2000.

Saturday Evening Post, "The Stokes Family Saga," May 2000.

Cory SerVaas and Patrick Perry, "Coronary Gene Therapy: Restoring Hope and Lives," *Saturday Evening Post*, May 2000.

E. M. Swift and Don Yeager, "Unnatural Selection," *Sports Illustrated*, May 14, 2001.

Larry Thompson, "Human Gene Therapy: Harsh Lessons, High Hopes." *FDA Consumer*, September 2000.

Helen Thorpe, "Cancer Patience," *Texas Monthly*, January 1997.

Meredith Wadman, "Can Gene Therapy Cure This Child?" *Fortune*, May 1, 2000.

Jeff Wheelwright, "Betting on Designer Genes," *Smithsonian*, January 2001.

Internet Sources

Emilie R. Bergeson, "The Ethics of Gene Therapy," 1997. www.ndsu.nodak/edu/instruct/mcclean/plsc431/students/bergeson.htm. Student essay from North Dakota State University at Fargo providing extensive background and overview of gene therapy, including technical aspects and pro and con arguments.

Kennedy Institute of Ethics, Georgetown University, "Human Gene Therapy, Scope Note 24," February 2000. www.georgetown.edu/research/nrcbl/scopenotes/sn24.htm. Overview, including background, techniques, candidate diseases, history, arguments in favor of and against gene therapy, and organizational statements and policies.

Websites

Institute for Human Gene Therapy. www.med.upenn.edu/ihgt. Includes statement on death of Jesse

Gelsinger and research briefs on treatments for cystic fibrosis, muscular dystrophy, and other diseases.

National Human Genome Research Institute (NHGRI). www.nhgri.nih.gov. Describes the Human Genome Project, its background, and its ethical, legal, and social implications.

Oak Ridge National Laboratory. www.ornl.gov/hgmis/ medicine/genetherapy.html. General article on gene therapy, with references to other articles.

WORKS CONSULTED

Books

Walter Bodmer and Robin McKie, *The Book of Man*. New York: Scribner's, 1994. History of human genetics, focusing on recent advances such as the Human Genome Project.

Ruth Hubbard and Elijah Wald, *Exploding the Gene Myth: How Genetic Information Is Produced and Manipulated by Scientists, Physicians, Employers, Insurance Companies, Educators, and Law Enforcers*. Boston: Beacon Press, 1997. Includes material that questions excessive emphasis on the role of genes in determining human personality and behavior and throws doubt on the ethics of most alteration of human genes.

N. R. Lemoine, ed., *Understanding Gene Therapy*. Oxford, UK: Bios Scientific Publishers, 1999. Fairly technical book on current gene-therapy experiments and different types of vectors (carriers) for therapeutic genes.

Joseph Levine and David Suzuki, *The Secret of Life*. Boston: WGBH Educational Foundation, 1993. Describes what scientists have learned about the genes that shape a human being.

Gregory Stock and John Campbell, eds., *Engineering the Human Germline: An Exploration of the Science and Ethics of Altering the Genes We Pass to Our Children*. New York: Oxford Press, 2000. Papers from a symposium held in 1998 at the University of California at Los Angeles; presents a mostly positive view of germline gene alteration.

Periodicals

Tom Abate, "Alameda Biotech Firm Boosts Gene Therapy," *San Francisco Chronicle*, December 7, 1999.

———, "Death Reports Spark No Cries for Demise of Gene Therapy Studies," *San Francisco Chronicle*, November 8, 1999.

———, "Genentech's Heart Drug Disappoints," *San Francisco Chronicle*, February 19, 1999.

———, "Possible Leap Forward for Hemophiliacs," *San Francisco Chronicle*, April 12, 1999.

———, "Race to Heal a Broken Heart," *San Francisco Chronicle*, February 15, 1999.

E. W. F. W. Alton, "Cationic Lipid-Mediated CFTR Gene Transfer to the Lungs and Nose of Patients with Cystic Fibrosis: A Double-Blind Placebo-Controlled Trial," *Journal of the American Medical Association*, June 2, 1999.

W. French Anderson, "The Best of Times, the Worst of Times," *Science*, April 28, 2000.

———, "A Cure That May Cost Us Ourselves," *Newsweek*, January 1, 2000.

———, "Gene Therapy," *Scientific American*, September 1995.

Associated Press, "Gene Therapy Used with Drugs Shrinks Tumors," *San Francisco Chronicle*, August 2, 2000.

Virginia Barbour, "The Balance of Risk and Benefit in Gene-Therapy Trials," *Lancet*, January 29, 2000.

Sharon Begley, "Designer Babies," *Newsweek*, November 9, 1998.

———, "Into the Gene Pool," *Newsweek*, December 28, 1998.

BioWorld Week, "FDA: Companies Slow to Respond to Requests," April 9, 2001.

BioWorld Week, "NIH Group Makes Gene Therapy Recommendation," June 12, 2000.

BioWorld Week, "Senate Eyes Protection of Gene Therapy Subjects," May 29, 2000.

R. Michael Blaese, "Gene Therapy for Cancer," *Scientific American,* June 1997.

Jane Bradbury, "Extensions Planned for Adenovirus-Associated Viruses," *Lancet,* May 6, 2000.

Business Week,"Gene Researchers, Hold Your Hype," April 3, 2000.

Business Week, "One Death in 5,000 Shouldn't Doom Gene Therapy," December 13, 1999.

Business Week, "Score One for Gene Therapy," May 8, 2000.

James Butcher, "New Hope for Gene Therapy?" *Lancet,* August 5, 2000.

———, "Will Gene Therapy for Parkinson's Disease Prove Viable?" *Lancet,* October 28, 2000.

Angie Cannon, "Humility at the Frontier," *U.S. News & World Report,* December 20, 1999.

Terence Chea, "Gene Therapy's Hot Seat: Ignoring Skeptics, GenVec Forges Ahead with Drug Development," *Washington Post,* February 20, 2001.

Christian Century, "Study Cites Dangers in Modifying Genes," October 25, 2000.

Dinesh D'Souza and Ronald Bailey, "Our Biotech Future—An Exchange," *National Review,* March 5, 2001.

Carol Featherstone, "Old Hopes and New Horizons for Treating Cystic Fibrosis," *Lancet,* June 1, 1996.

Joannie Fischer, "Passing on Perfection," *U.S. News & World Report,* October 2, 2000.

Theodore Friedmann, "Overcoming the Obstacles to Gene Therapy," *Scientific American,* June 1997.

———, "Principles for Human Gene Therapy Studies," *Science,* March 24, 2000.

Tanya Gregory and Nelson A. Wivel, "Clinical Applications of Molecular Medicine," *Patient Care,* November 15, 1998.

Trisha Gura, "Repairing the Genome's Spelling Mistakes," *Science,* July 16, 1999.

John Harris, "Intimations of Immortality," *Science,* April 7, 2000.

Leon Jaroff, "Success Stories," *Time,* January 11, 1999.

Leon R. Kass, "The Moral Meaning of Genetic Technology," *Commentary,* September 1999.

Lancet, "Gene Therapy Under Cloud," January 29, 2000.

Marilynn Larkin and Jane Bradbury, "Promising Results Reported for Lung Cancer Gene Therapy," *Lancet,* September 7, 1996.

Michael McCarthy, "FDA Puts US Gene-Therapy Trial on Hold," *Lancet,* March 11, 2000.

———, "US FDA Rejects Defence of Gene-Therapy Trial," *Lancet,* March 18, 2000.

———, "Vascular Gene Therapy Studies Show Promise," *Lancet,* November 15, 1997.

Eliot Marshall, "One Less Hoop for Gene Therapy," *Science,* July 29, 1994.

Mary Midgley, "Biotechnology and Monstrosity: Why We Should Pay Attention to the 'Yuk Factor,'" *Hastings Center Report,* September 2000.

Julie Ann Miller, "Lessons from Asilomar," *Science News,* February 23, 1985.

Lance Morrow, "How to Mend a Broken Heart," *Time,* November 22, 1999.

Deborah Nelson and Rick Weiss, "Gene-Experiment Deaths Confirmed by Researchers," *Washington Post.* Reprinted in *San Francisco Chronicle,* November 3, 1999.

———, "Penn Researchers Sued in Gene Therapy Death," *Washington Post,* September 19, 2000.

Newsday, "Hemophilia Gene Therapy Shows Promise." Reprinted in *San Francisco Chronicle,* March 1, 2000.

Amy Otchet, "The Dangers of Laissez Faire Eugenics," *UNESCO Courier,* September 1999.

Sarah Ramsay, "Investigators Report Gene-Therapy Success for Chronic Myocardial Ischaemia," *Lancet,* September 2, 2000.

Paul Recer, "Researchers Blamed for Death," *San Francisco Chronicle,* December 9, 1999.

Leslie Roberts, "A Promising Experiment Ends in Tragedy," *U.S. News & World Report,* October 11, 1999.

San Francisco Chronicle, "Gene Trials Show Few Violations, FDA Audit Says," April 9, 2001.

San Francisco Chronicle, "Health Officials Admit Oversight in Gene Studies," February 2, 2000.

San Francisco Chronicle, "New Rules Aim to Protect Gene Therapy Patients," March 8, 2000.

San Francisco Chronicle, "New Theory on Cause of Gene-Therapy Death," December 2, 1999.

Science News, "Gene Therapy Advances Go to the Heart," November 28, 1998.

N. Seppa, "Therapy Pits Useful Gene Against Tumor," *Science News,* May 15, 1999.

Robert Sikorski and Richard Peters, "Treating with HIV," *Science,* November 20, 1998.

S. Simpson, "Gene Injections Stem Clotting Disorder," *Science News,* January 16, 1999.

Joan Stephenson, "Gene Therapy Trials Show Clinical Efficacy," *Journal of the American Medical Association,* February 2, 2000.

Sheryl Gay Stolberg, "Gene Therapy Institute Scaled Back After Patient's Death," *New York Times.* Reprinted in *San Francisco Chronicle,* May 25, 2000.

Helen Thorpe, "Jack Roth: He's Helping Solve One of Medicine's Biggest Mysteries: Cancer. It's All in the Genes," *Texas Monthly,* September 1998.

Ulysses Torassa, "Gene Therapy Could Help Hemophiliacs," *San Francisco Chronicle,* December 5, 2000.

John Travis, "Cystic Fibrosis Controversy," *Science News*, May 10, 1997.

———, "Inner Strength," *Science News*, March 14, 1998.

Virus Weekly, "Gene Therapy Shown to Protect and Reverse Debilitating Effects in Pre-Clinical Studies," November 7, 2000.

Washington Post, "Apology for Gene Therapy Death." Reprinted in *San Francisco Chronicle*, December 10, 1999.

Washington Post, "FDA Warns Doctor Who Led Fatal Gene-Therapy Experiment." Reprinted in *San Francisco Chronicle*, May 3, 2000.

Washington Post, "Gene Therapy Hearing Stalls over Disclosure." Reprinted in *San Francisco Chronicle*, December 11, 1999.

Washington Post, "More Gene-Therapy Trials Halted over Safety Fears." Reprinted in *San Francisco Chronicle*, February 8, 2000.

Washington Post, "Probe of Death Prompts Halt to Penn's Gene Tests." Reprinted in *San Francisco Chronicle*, January 22, 2000.

Ralph R. Weichselbaum and Donald Kufe, "Gene Therapy of Cancer," *Lancet*, May 17, 1997.

Rick Weiss, "FDA Seeks to Penalize Gene Scientist," *Washington Post*, December 12, 2000.

———, "Gene Therapy Benefits Cited; Study Suggests Diseased Heart Cells Renewed; Doubts Remain," *Washington Post*, August 29, 2000.

———, "New Rule for Gene Therapy Tests Proposed," *Washington Post*, January 18, 2001.

———, "NIH Panel Backs Easing of Gene Therapy Rules," *Washington Post*, June 30, 2000.

———, "Two Successes with Gene Therapy," *Washington Post*. Reprinted in *San Francisco Chronicle*, April 28, 2000.

Rick Weiss and Deborah Nelson, "Penn Settles Gene Therapy Suit," *Washington Post*, November 4, 2000.

Edward O. Wilson, "A World of Immortal Men," *Esquire,* May 1999.

Savio L. C. Woo, "Gene Therapy Researchers React to Field's Pitfalls and Promises," *FDA Consumer,* September 2000.

Seppo Yla-Herttuala and John F. Martin, "Cardiovascular Gene Therapy," *Lancet,* January 15, 2000.

Esmail D. Zanjani and W. French Anderson, "Prospects for in Utero Human Gene Therapy," *Science,* September 24, 1999.

Internet Sources

American Society of Gene Therapy, "Position/Policy Statement on Financial Conflict of Interest in Clinical Research." www.asgt.org/policy.

Donald M. Bruce, "Gene Therapy," Society, Religion, and Technology Project, Church of Scotland, 1996. http://dspace.dial.pipex.com/srtscot/genthpy1.htm.

Cystic Fibrosis Foundation, "Gene Therapy and Cystic Fibrosis," March 30, 2001. www.cff.org/publications 03.htm.

Kevin C. Kelley, "The Hope and Hype of Hemophilia Gene Therapy," *Parent Exchange Newsletter*, February 1999. www.kelleycom.com/pengene.htm.

Muscular Dystrophy Association, "Gene Therapy Entering the Clinic," *MDA/Quest,* August 1999. www.mdausa.org/publications/Quest/gt-lmenu. html.

———, "New Hope for Gene Therapy of DMD, BMD Using AAV Vectors," *MDA/Quest,* August 2000. www.mdausa.org/publications/Quest/q74resup. html#newhope.

Stuart H. Orkin and Arno G. Motulsky, "Report and Recommendations of the Panel to Assess the NIH Investment in Research on Gene Therapy," NIH website, December 1995. www.nih.gov/news/panelrep. html.

PR Newswire, "Cell Genesys Reports Interim Findings for AIDS Gene Therapy Clinical Trials," February 5, 1998. www.aegis.com/news/pr/1998/PR980221.html.

Steven A. Rosenberg, "The Development of Cancer Vaccines," National Cancer Institute website. www.cancerresearch.org/cancervaccines2000/steven_rosenberg.html.

Science Daily, "Gene Therapy Revives 'Hibernating' Heart Muscle," August 29, 2000. www.sciencedaily.com/releases/2000/08/000829080409.htm.

Science Daily, "Gene Therapy Halts HIV Replication in Cells from Infected Patients, According to the Children's Hospital of Philadelphia," February 21, 2000. www.sciencedaily.com/releases/2000/02/00216122207.htm.

Signals, "High Noon for Gene Therapy," July 23, 1999. www.signalsmag.com/signalsmag.nsf/657b06742b5748e888256570005cba01/7798e274f16aeb28882567b5006537d6?OpenDocument.

University of Toronto students, "Glioblastoma Treatments," University of Toronto website. http://dragon.zoo.utoronto.ca/~J01T0701C/gttreat.htm.

———, "Hemophilia Gene Therapy: Issues and Perspectives," University of Toronto website, March 2001. http://dragon.zoo.utoronto.ca/~J01T0301C/index2.html.

———, "Interview with Dr. S. Mackenzie of Trillium Health Care Centre and Dr. Bouffet," University of Toronto website, February 5, 2001. http://dragon.zoo.utoronto.ca/~J01T0201B/inter1.htm.

INDEX

PICTURE CREDITS

About the Author

Lisa Yount earned a bachelor's degree with honors in English and creative writing from Stanford University. She has a lifelong interest in biology and medicine. She has been a professional writer for thirty-five years, producing educational materials, magazine articles, and thirty books for young adults and adults. Her books for Lucent include *Issues in Biomedical Ethics*, *Cancer*, and *Epidemics*. She lives in El Cerrito, California, with her husband, a large library, and several cats.